Blood Test Breakdown

I0422826

Understanding Your Medical Results

Book design by Lisa Buchanan
Cover design by Lisa Buchanan

This page left intentionally blank.

Dear Reader,

Have you ever stared at a blood test report filled with numbers and abbreviations, wondering what it all means? You're not alone! Blood tests, while crucial for understanding our health, can often feel like a cryptic code. But fear not! This book, "Blood Test Breakdown: Understanding Your Medical Results," is your guide to cracking that code.

Blood tests are the unsung heroes of preventive healthcare. They offer a window into our inner workings, revealing vital information about our overall health. Imagine them as a secret language your body uses to communicate potential issues before they escalate into bigger problems. By analyzing various components in your blood, like cholesterol and enzymes, doctors can identify risk factors for diseases like heart disease, diabetes, and liver problems. Early detection is key – it allows for timely intervention and treatment, often preventing the development of more serious conditions.

But blood tests are more than just crystal balls for future health woes. They also play a vital role in managing existing conditions and monitoring the effectiveness of treatment. Think of them as a progress report on your health journey. For example, someone with diabetes might rely on regular blood tests to track their blood sugar levels and adjust their medication accordingly. Similarly, chemotherapy patients might undergo frequent blood tests to monitor their white blood cell count and ensure treatment isn't causing harmful side effects. In essence, blood tests provide valuable insights that may not be readily apparent through symptoms alone. By understanding these results, you'll be empowered to take a proactive approach to your health. Whether it's making lifestyle changes to improve your cholesterol levels or working with your doctor to refine your medication regimen based on your blood sugar readings, the knowledge gleaned from blood tests equips you to make informed decisions about your well-being.

This book is your roadmap to navigating the world of blood tests. We'll delve into the common tests, explain what the results mean, and equip you with the knowledge to have a more informed conversation with your doctor. So, grab your metaphorical magnifying glass, and let's embark on this journey of understanding your health through the power of blood tests!

Sincerely,

Lisa Buchanan

Author Bio

Lisa Buchanan is a passionate advocate for health literacy. After spending eleven years at the world's leading medical blood laboratory, she witnessed firsthand the power of understanding your blood test results. Lisa has dedicated herself to translating complex medical jargon into clear, easy-to-understand language.

Feeling lost when you receive your blood test reports? You're not alone! Packed with technical terms and seemingly random numbers, blood tests can be intimidating. But what if you could understand them with ease?

In this comprehensive guide, Lisa Buchanan, a veteran of the world's top medical blood lab, empowers you to take control of your health. Forget the confusion! 'Blood Test Breakdown' explains everything you need to know about routine blood work in clear, concise language.

Thank You!

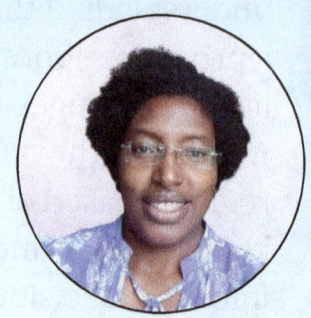

Lisa Buchanan

Author

TABLE OF CONTENTS

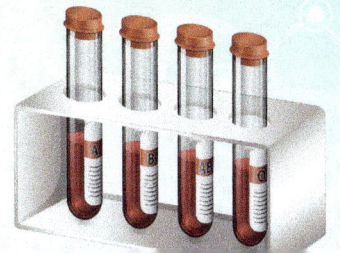

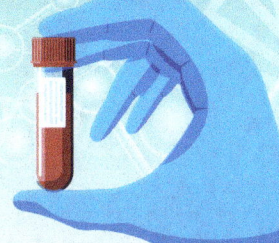

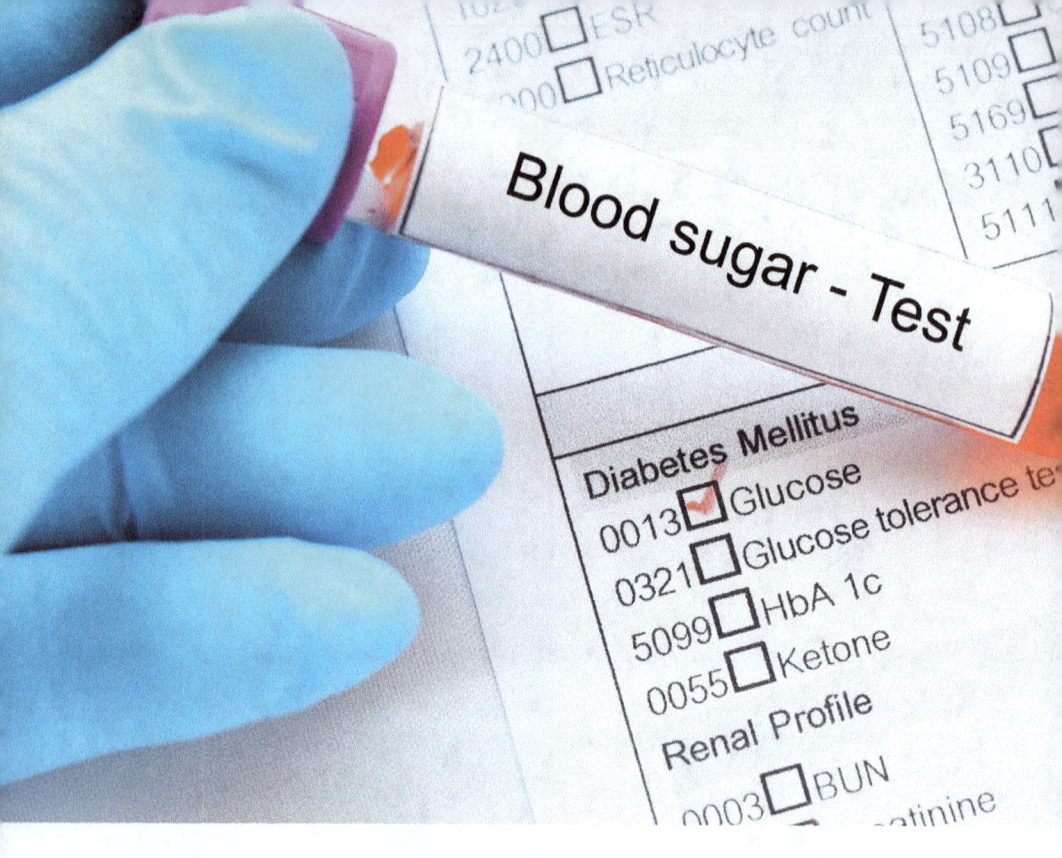

Chapter 1:

Introduction to Medical Blood Tests

The Importance of Blood Tests

Blood tests are crucial tools that provide vital information about your overall health and well-being. Understanding the results of these tests can help you and your healthcare provider make informed decisions about your health.

One of the key reasons why blood tests are so important is that they can **detect potential health issues before they become serious problems.** By analyzing the levels of various substances in your blood, such as cholesterol, glucose, and various enzymes, healthcare providers can identify risk factors for conditions like heart disease, diabetes, and liver disease. Early detection allows for timely intervention and treatment, which can often prevent the development of more serious health issues.

In addition to detecting potential health problems, blood tests are also used to monitor existing conditions and track the effectiveness of treatment. For example, individuals with diabetes may need regular blood tests to monitor their blood sugar levels and adjust their treatment plan accordingly. Similarly, individuals undergoing chemotherapy may require frequent blood tests to monitor their white blood cell count and ensure that their treatment is not causing harmful side effects.

Overall, blood tests provide valuable insights into your health that may not be apparent through symptoms alone. By understanding the results of these tests, you can take proactive steps to maintain or improve your health.

Hematological ~~ry Report~~ Co

Name: John Smithw
Date: 09/12
Physician: Dr. Jones

Lab		Range
WBC	5100K/mL	4-10K/mL
Hgb	15.5g/dL	3.5-17,5 g/dL
HgbA1c	6.5%	7.5 %
Hct	41.00%	
BC	4.9 x 106 cells/mL	106 cell
u	75 mg/dL	/dL
l	8 mg/dL	7-1
l	1.0 mg/dL	0.5-1.2 mg/dL
	140 mm/hr	0-20 mm/hr

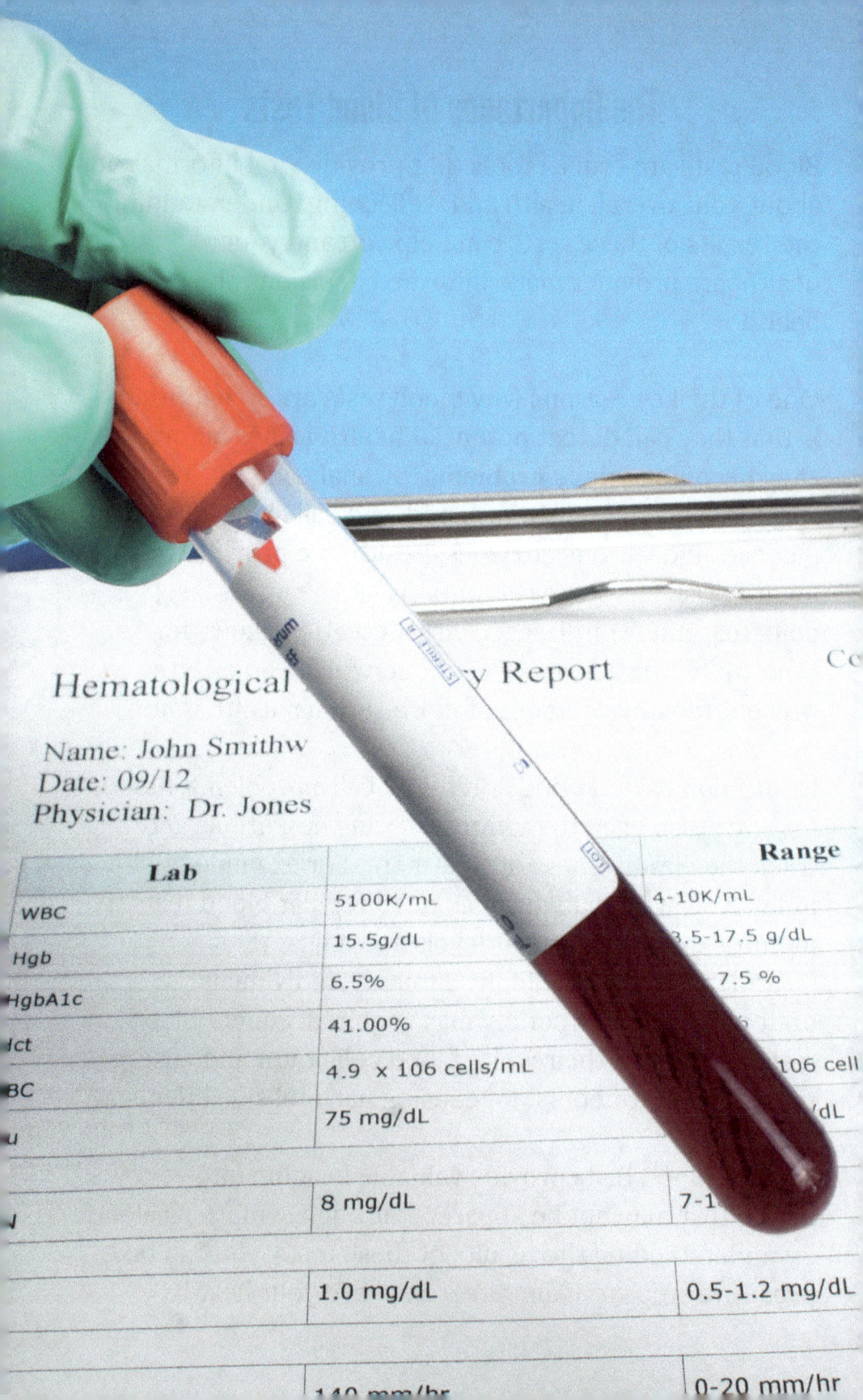

Whether it's making lifestyle changes to lower your cholesterol levels or adjusting your medication regimen based on your blood sugar levels, the information provided by blood tests can help you make informed decisions about your health and well-being

Color Coded Blood Tubes

Ever noticed those vials with colorful caps when you get blood drawn? They're not just there for fun! Those colors actually have a "secret code" that doctors and nurses use. Each color tells them what's inside the tube and what kind of test will be done on your blood.

Think of the tubes like tiny containers with special ingredients. Some ingredients stop your blood from clotting, like putting a pause button on it. Others help separate the different parts of your blood, like the cells swimming in a liquid called plasma. The colored caps help everyone remember which ingredient is in which tube.

For example, a red-top tube might have a clot activator inside. This means it lets your blood clot normally, and doctors can then analyze the liquid leftover after the clot forms, called serum. This serum is useful for tests like checking your immunity or hormones. On the other hand, a purple-top tube might have an anticoagulant, like a little roadblock, to prevent clotting. This keeps your blood cells from sticking together, which is important for tests that look at those cells themselves.

So next time you see those colorful tubes, remember, it's a secret code to help doctors get the most accurate information from your amazing blood!

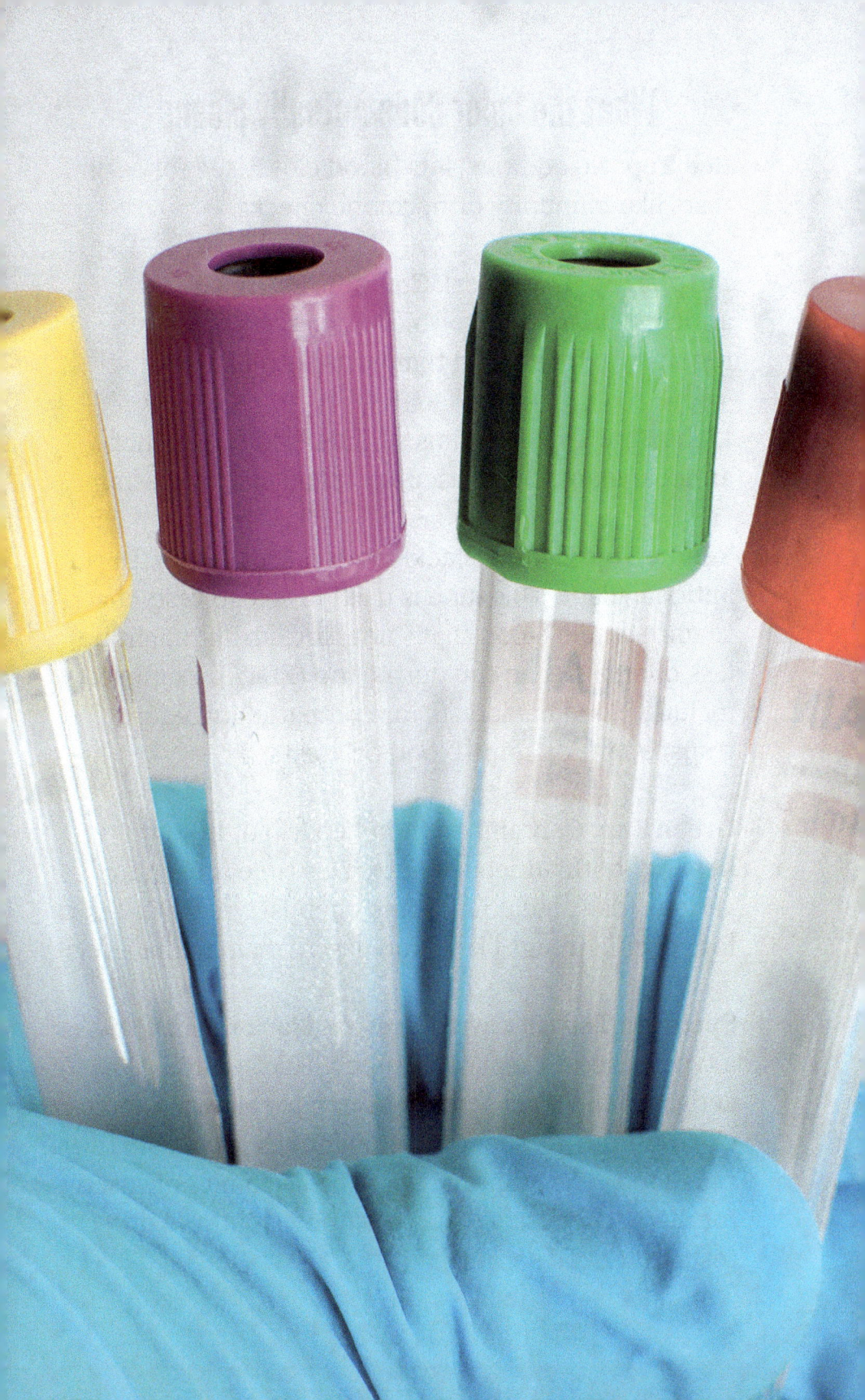

What the Color Code Actually Means

- **Red Top:** No additive, lets blood clot. Used for serum tests like immunity or hormone checks.

- **Purple Top (Lavender):** Contains EDTA, an anticoagulant. Used for blood cell tests or tests requiring whole blood that isn't clotted.

- **Light Blue Top:** Contains sodium citrate, another anticoagulant. Often used for blood clotting tests.

- **Yellow Top:** Contains acid citrate dextrose (ACD), an anticoagulant. This tube is used for blood tests that require whole blood that's not clotted, but might be less common than the purple top (EDTA). Examples include blood bank tests for compatibility before transfusions or some blood cell tests.

- **Green Top:** Contains sodium heparin or lithium heparin, both anticoagulants. This tube is used for various tests, including some chemistry tests or tests for specific things like blood gases or ammonia levels

- **Speckled Top (Red with Gray or Black flecks):** This is a type of serum separator tube (SST). It contains a clot activator and a gel. The clot activator allows blood to clot, and the gel separates the liquid serum from the red blood cells after clotting. This is commonly used for many chemistry tests, hormone tests, and other tests that need serum.

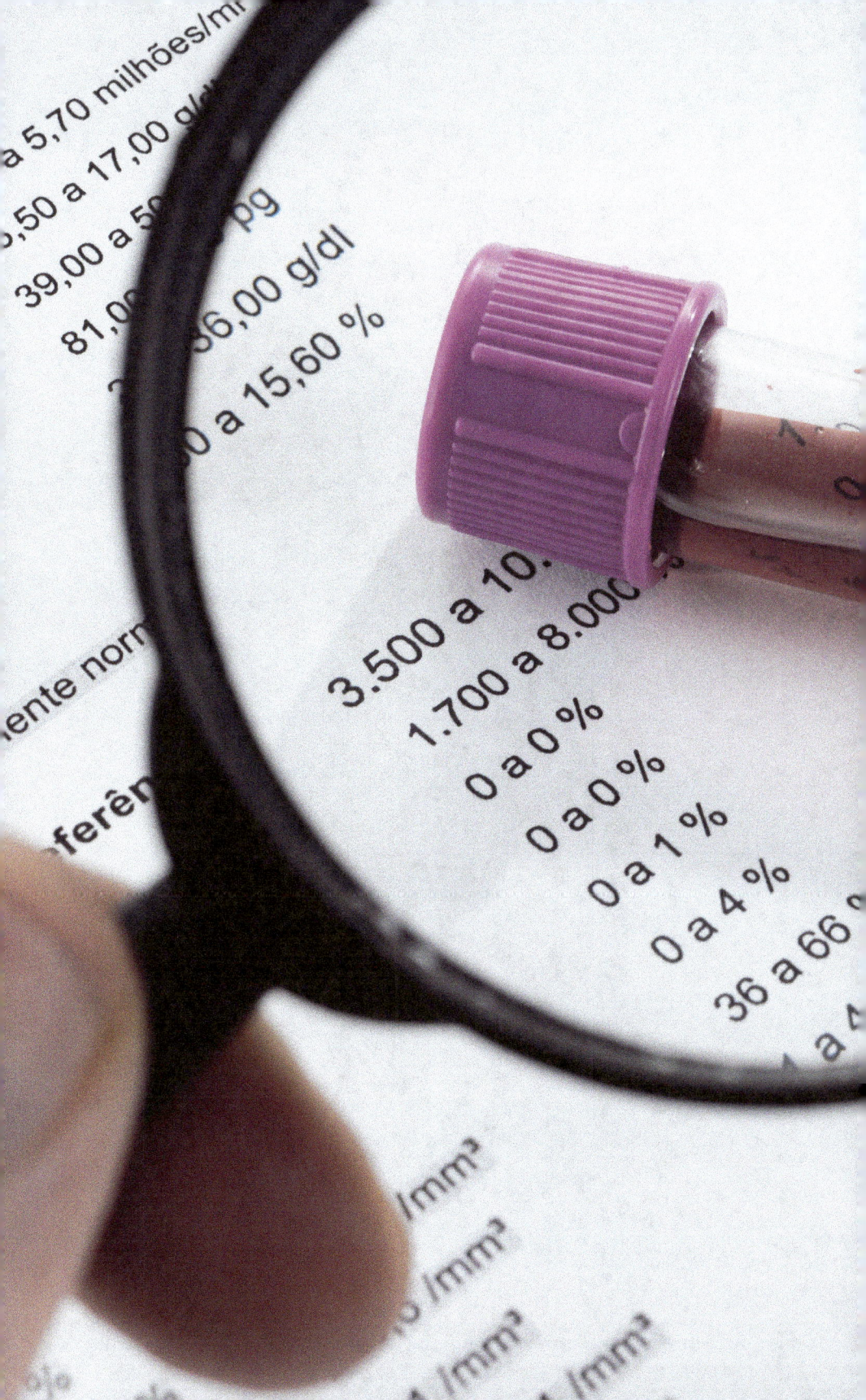

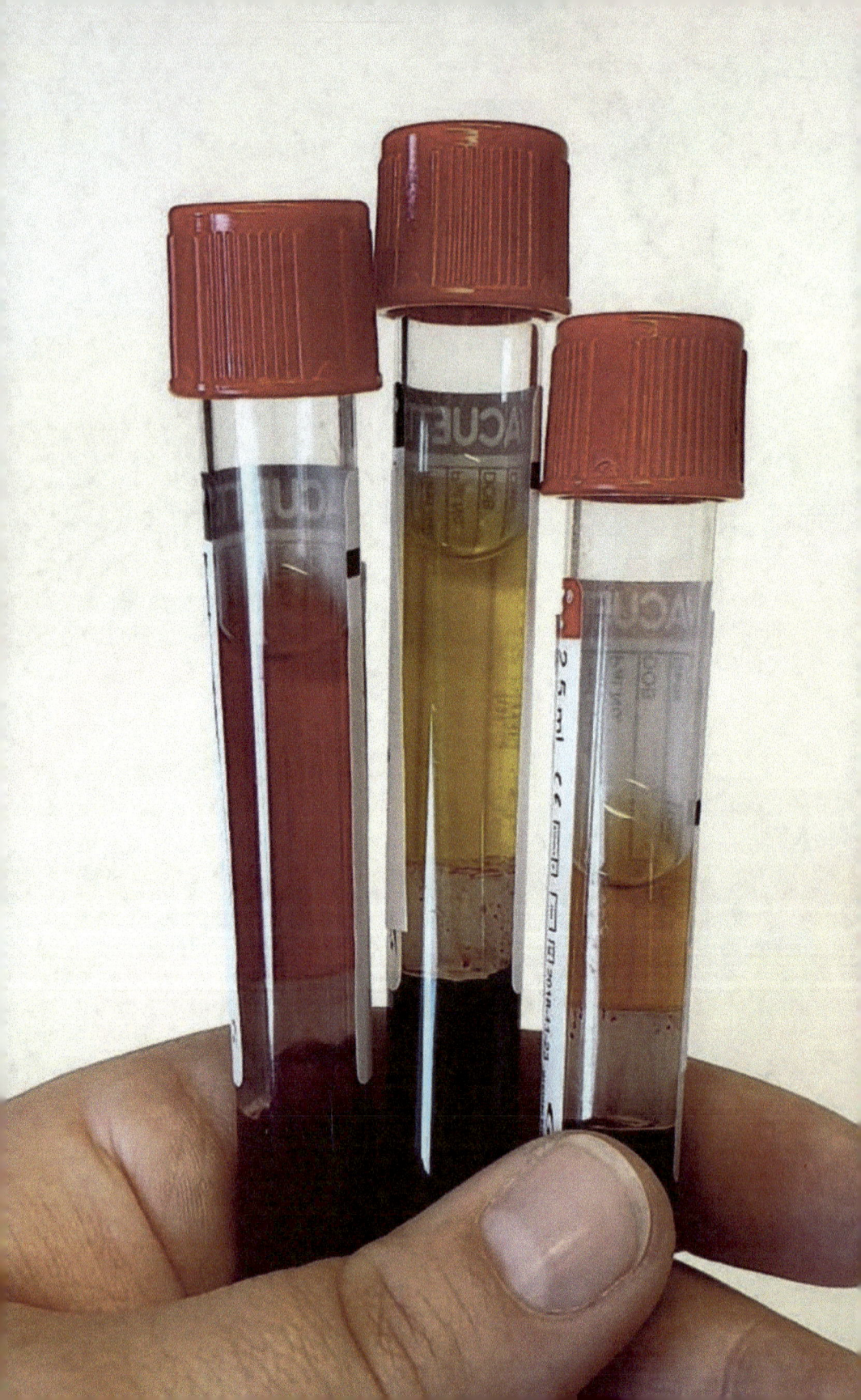

Common Types of Blood Tests

In order to fully understand your overall health and potential medical concerns, it is important to have a basic understanding of the common types of blood tests that your doctor may order. These tests are essential for diagnosing various health conditions, monitoring the effectiveness of treatments, and assessing your overall well-being.

One of the most common types of blood tests is the complete blood count (CBC), which provides information about your red blood cells, white blood cells, and platelets. This test can help identify conditions such as anemia, infections, and clotting disorders.

Another important blood test is the basic metabolic panel (BMP), which measures your blood glucose levels, electrolyte levels, and kidney function. Abnormal results on this test can point to issues such as diabetes, dehydration, or kidney disease.

The lipid panel is another common blood test that measures your cholesterol levels. High cholesterol levels can increase your risk of heart disease and stroke, so it is important to monitor these levels regularly.

Additionally, the liver function test (LFT) can provide valuable information about the health of your liver. Abnormal results on this test can indicate liver damage, hepatitis, or other liver disorders.

It is important to note that these are just a few examples of the many types of blood tests that your doctor may

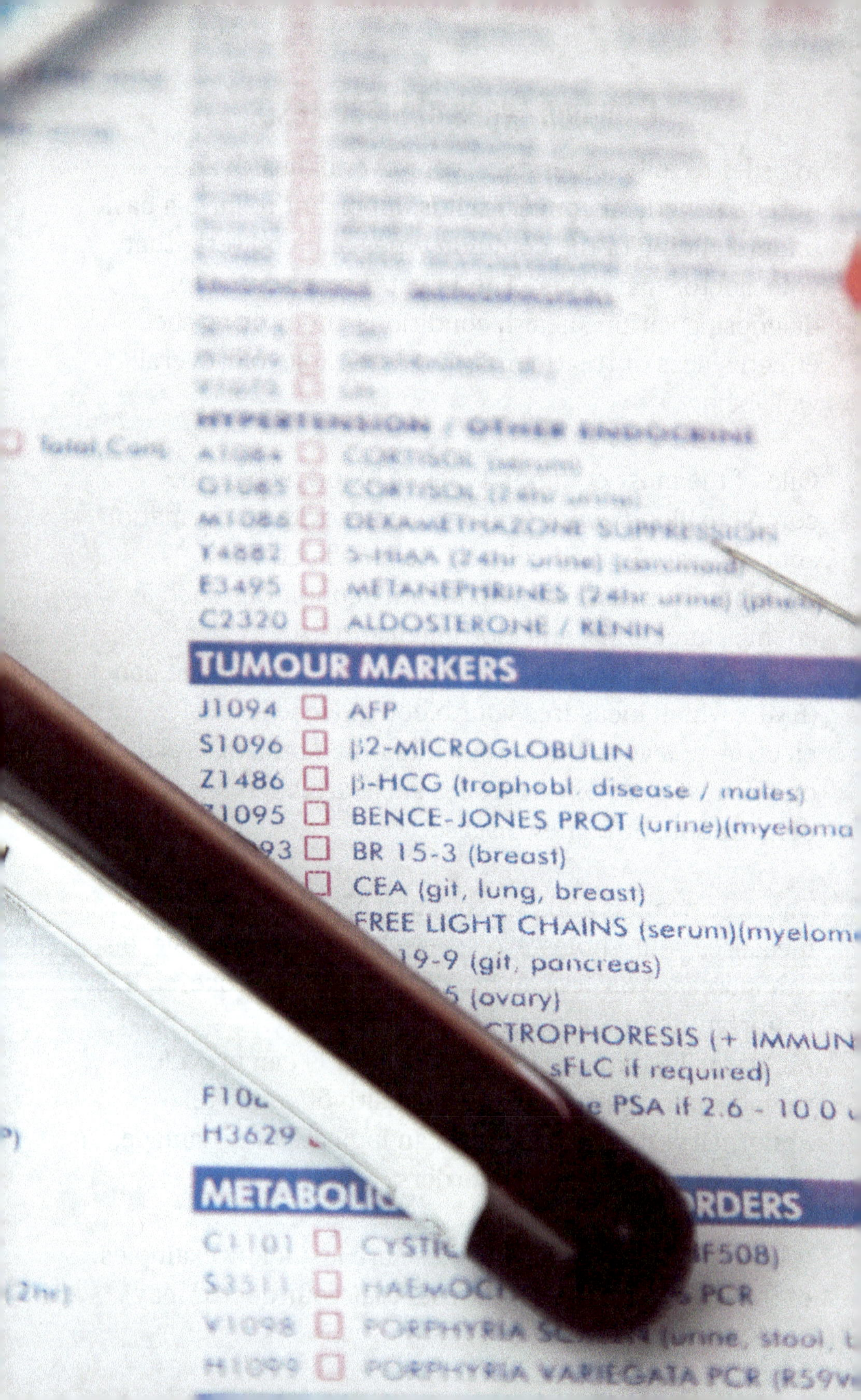

HYPERTENSION / OTHER ENDOCRINE

A1084 ☐ CORTISOL (serum)
G1085 ☐ CORTISOL (24hr urine)
M1086 ☐ DEXAMETHAZONE SUPPRESSION
Y4882 ☐ 5-HIAA (24hr urine) (carcinoid)
E3495 ☐ METANEPHRINES (24hr urine) (phae
C2320 ☐ ALDOSTERONE / RENIN

TUMOUR MARKERS

J1094 ☐ AFP
S1096 ☐ β2-MICROGLOBULIN
Z1486 ☐ β-HCG (trophobl. disease / males)
Z1095 ☐ BENCE-JONES PROT (urine)(myeloma
...93 ☐ BR 15-3 (breast)
☐ CEA (git, lung, breast)
FREE LIGHT CHAINS (serum)(myelome
...9-9 (git, pancreas)
...5 (ovary)
CTROPHORESIS (+ IMMUN
sFLC if required)
e PSA if 2.6 - 10.0

F10...
H3629

METABOLIC ...ORDERS

C1101 ☐ CYSTI... (...F508)
S3511 ☐ HAEMOC... PCR
V1098 ☐ PORPHYRIA SCREEN (urine, stool, ...)
H1099 ☐ PORPHYRIA VARIEGATA PCR (R59...

(2hr)

order. By understanding the purpose of these tests and what they can reveal about your health, you can be better

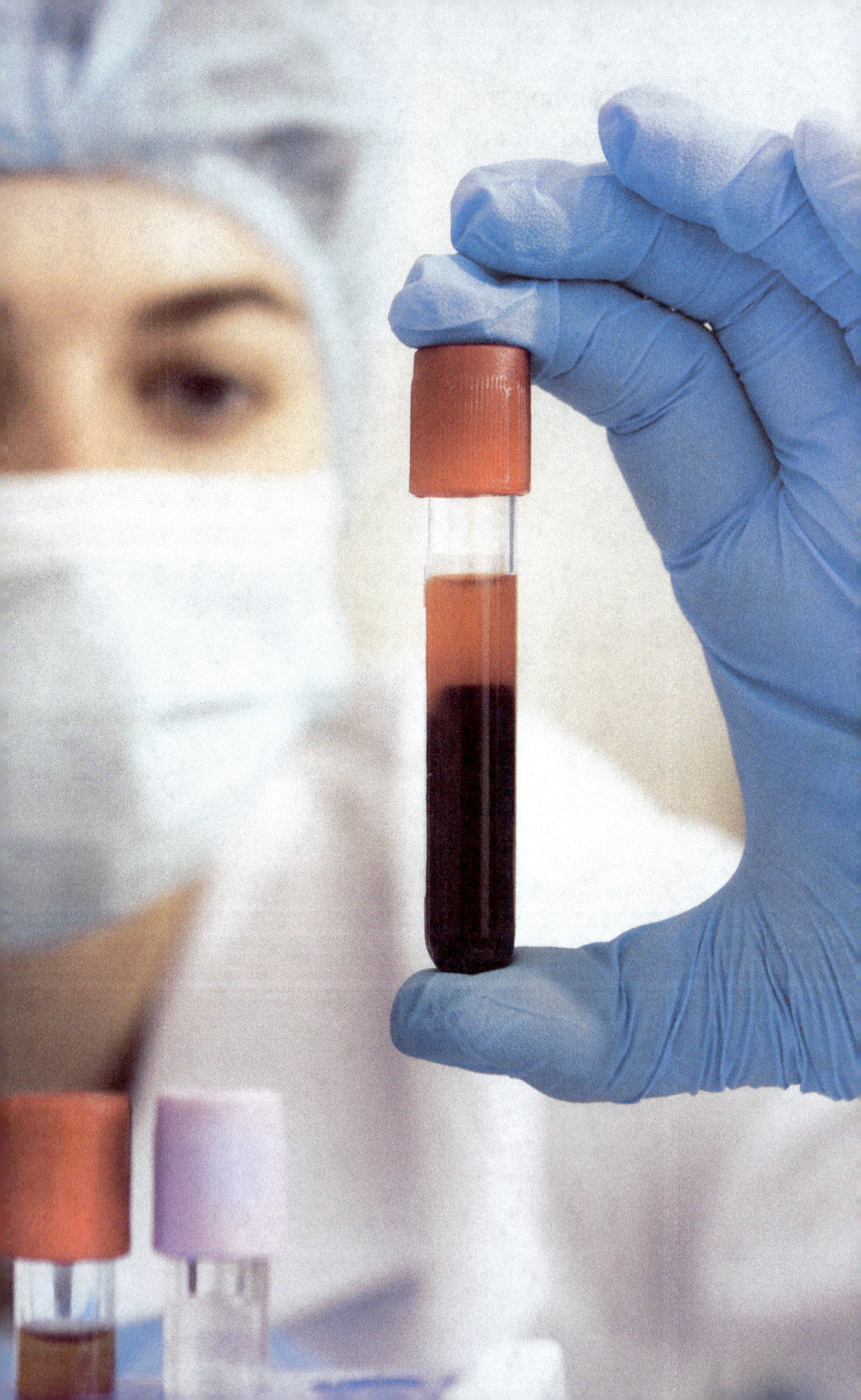

How Blood Tests are Administered

Blood tests are an essential part of understanding your overall health and well-being. Administering a blood test may seem like a complex process, but it is actually quite simple. In this subchapter, we will break down how blood tests are administered so that you can have a better understanding of what to expect when you go in for testing.

First, it is important to note that blood tests can be done in a variety of settings, including a doctor's office, clinic, or hospital. The process typically begins with a healthcare professional preparing you for the test by cleaning the area where the blood will be drawn. This is usually done with an alcohol swab to prevent infection.

Next, a tourniquet may be placed around your arm to help locate a vein for the blood draw. The healthcare professional will then use a needle to puncture the vein and collect a small sample of blood. This process may cause a slight pinch or sting, but it is generally well-tolerated by most individuals.

Once the blood sample is collected, it is typically sent to a laboratory for analysis. This is where the magic happens, as the blood is tested for various markers that can provide valuable insights into your health. These markers can indicate things like cholesterol levels, blood sugar levels, liver function, and more.

In conclusion, understanding how blood tests are

administered is an important step in taking control of your health. By knowing what to expect during the testing process, you can feel more confident and informed when discussing your results with your healthcare provider.

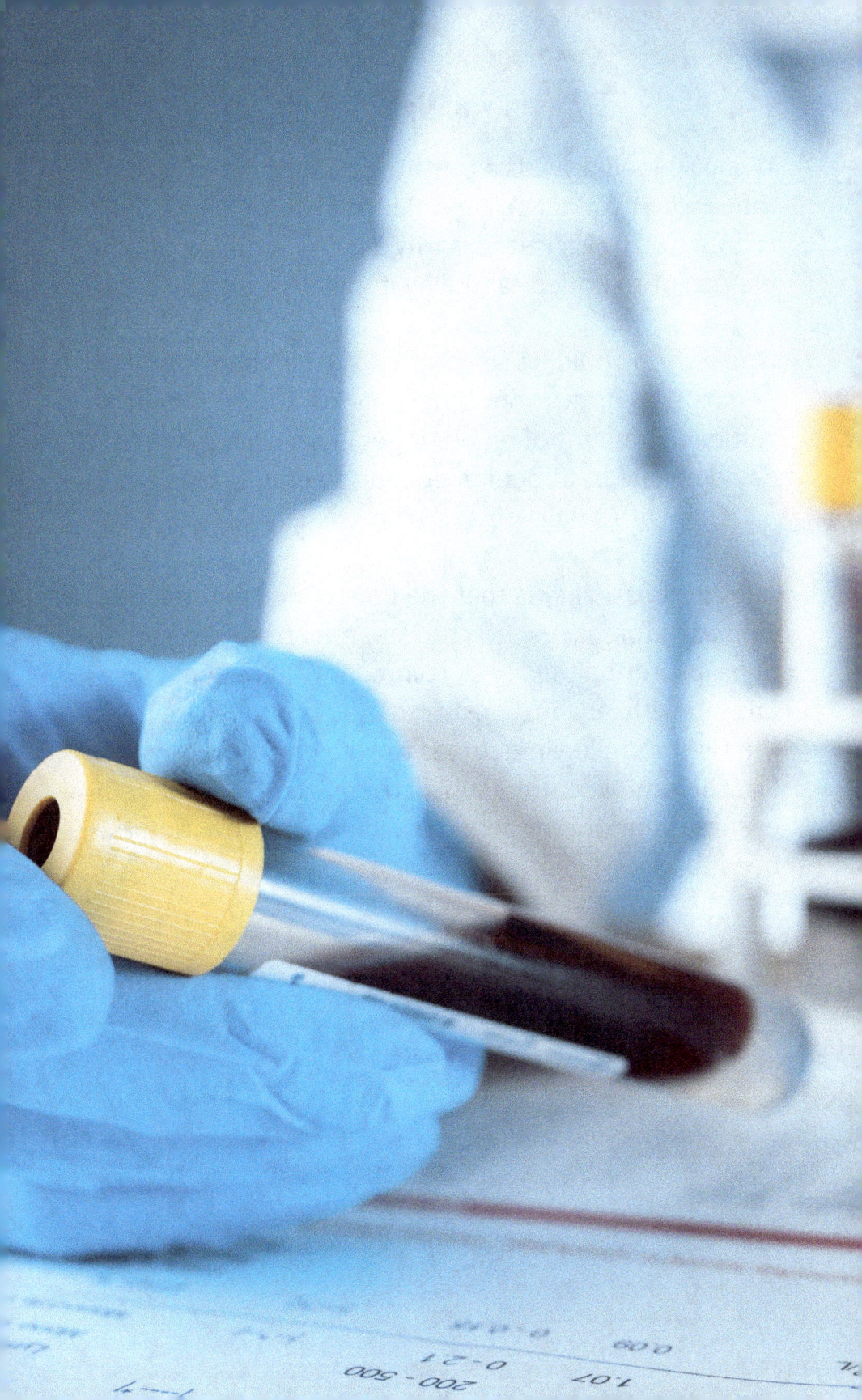

When You Need a Redraw

While a blood draw is a routine procedure, there are times when you might be called back in to have it redrawn. This isn't necessarily a cause for alarm, but it's important to understand why it might happen.

One reason could be simply that the phlebotomist, the person who draws your blood, wasn't able to obtain a sufficient amount of blood or get a clean sample. This could be due to difficulty locating a vein, especially for patients with small veins or who are dehydrated.

Another possibility is that the tube containing the blood clotted before it reached the lab, rendering the sample unusable for testing. Less commonly, there could be a mix-up with labeling, ensuring the right tests are run on the right sample. Sometimes the lab or the delivery driver lost the sample entirely. In all these cases, a quick redraw ensures your doctor gets the accurate information they need to assess your health.

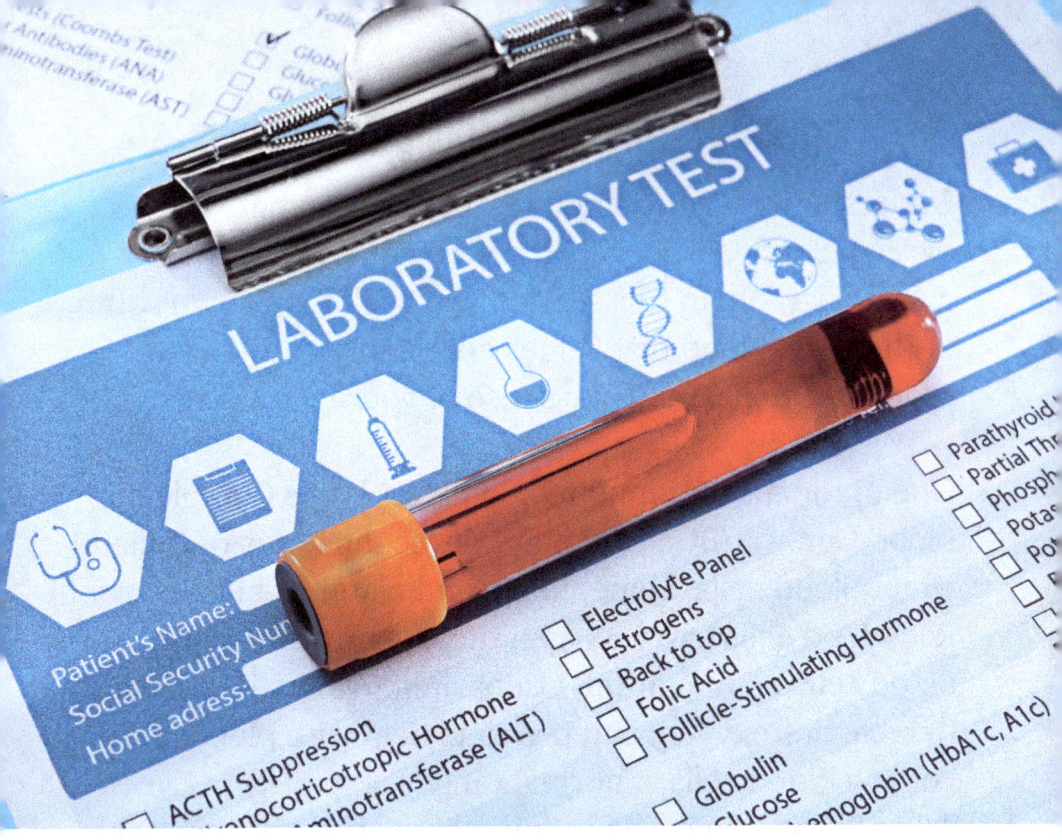

Chapter 2:

Understanding Blood Test Results

Interpreting Basic Blood Test Values

Understanding your blood test results can be overwhelming, especially if you're not familiar with medical jargon. In this section, we will break down some of the basic blood test values commonly seen on lab reports to help you make sense of your medical results.

One of the most common blood tests is the Complete Blood Count (CBC), which measures the levels of red and white blood cells, hemoglobin, and platelets in your blood. Red blood cells carry oxygen throughout your body, white blood cells help fight infections, hemoglobin is a protein that carries oxygen, and platelets help with blood clotting. For red blood cells, a normal range is typically between 4.2 to 5.4 million cells per microliter of blood. Low levels could indicate anemia, while high levels could be a sign of dehydration or lung disease. White blood cell counts are usually between 4,500 to 11,000 cells per microliter, with high levels indicating infection or inflammation.

Another important value to look at is your lipid panel, which measures cholesterol levels in your blood. High levels of LDL (bad) cholesterol and triglycerides can increase your risk of heart disease, while low levels of HDL (good) cholesterol can also be problematic. Understanding these basic blood test values can give you insight into your overall health and help you take proactive steps to improve your well-being. If you have any concerns about your results, don't hesitate to discuss them with your healthcare provider. Remember, knowledge is power when it comes to your health.

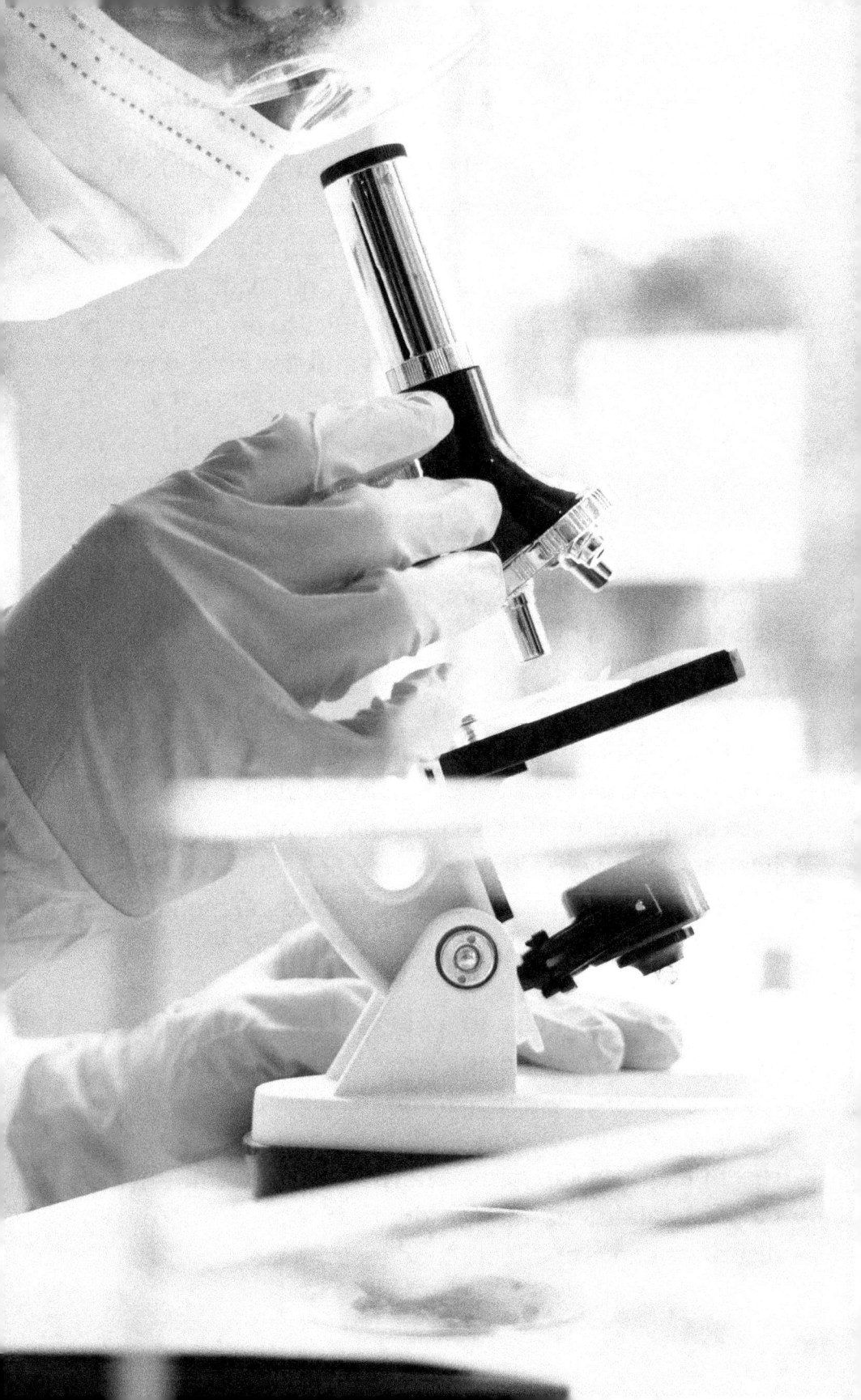

Factors that Affect Blood Test Results

Blood tests play a crucial role in monitoring our health and diagnosing various medical conditions. However, there are several factors that can affect the results of these tests, leading to inaccurate or misleading information. It is important for adults to be aware of these factors in order to better understand their blood test results.

One of the key factors that can impact blood test results is the timing of the test. Certain tests may need to be taken at specific times of the day or after fasting for accurate results. For example, fasting blood glucose levels can be affected by food intake, so it is important to fast for at least 8 hours before this test.

Another factor to consider is medication or supplements that you may be taking. Certain medications can interfere with blood test results, so it is important to inform your healthcare provider about any medications you are currently taking. This includes prescription medications, over-the-counter drugs, and herbal supplements.

Other factors that can affect blood test results include dehydration, stress, recent exercise, and underlying medical conditions. Dehydration can lead to elevated levels of certain substances in the blood, while stress and recent exercise can impact hormone levels. Underlying medical conditions such as kidney disease or thyroid disorders can also affect blood test results.

By understanding the various factors that can influence blood test results, adults can better interpret their medical results and work with their healthcare provider to ensure accurate diagnosis and treatment. It is important to communicate openly with your healthcare provider and follow any instructions for preparing for blood tests to ensure the most accurate results possible.

- [ ] Thyro
- [ ] Holter
- [ ] Protime
- [x] Cholest
- [x] Triglyce
- [x] HDL Cho

What Abnormal Results May Indicate

When you receive the results of your blood tests, it's important to understand what they mean. Abnormal results can indicate a variety of health issues that may require further investigation or treatment. Here are some common abnormal results and what they may indicate:

1. High cholesterol levels: High levels of cholesterol in your blood can increase your risk of heart disease and stroke. It may be a sign that you need to make dietary and lifestyle changes to improve your heart health.

2. Elevated blood sugar levels: High blood sugar levels can indicate diabetes or prediabetes. It's important to monitor your blood sugar levels regularly and work with your healthcare provider to manage your condition.

3. Abnormal liver function tests: Abnormal liver function tests may indicate liver damage or disease. Your healthcare provider may recommend additional tests to determine the cause of the abnormal results and develop a treatment plan.

4. Low levels of vitamin D: Low levels of vitamin D can lead to bone and muscle problems. Your healthcare provider may recommend supplements or dietary changes to increase your vitamin D levels.

5. Elevated white blood cell count: An elevated white blood cell count may indicate an infection or inflammation in your body. Your healthcare provider may recommend further testing to determine the cause of the elevated count.

Understanding what abnormal results may indicate is the first step in taking control of your health. If you receive abnormal results, don't panic. Instead, schedule a follow-up appointment with your healthcare provider to discuss your results and develop a plan of action. Remember, knowledge is power when it comes to your health.

Chapter 3:

Comprehensive Blood Test Breakdown

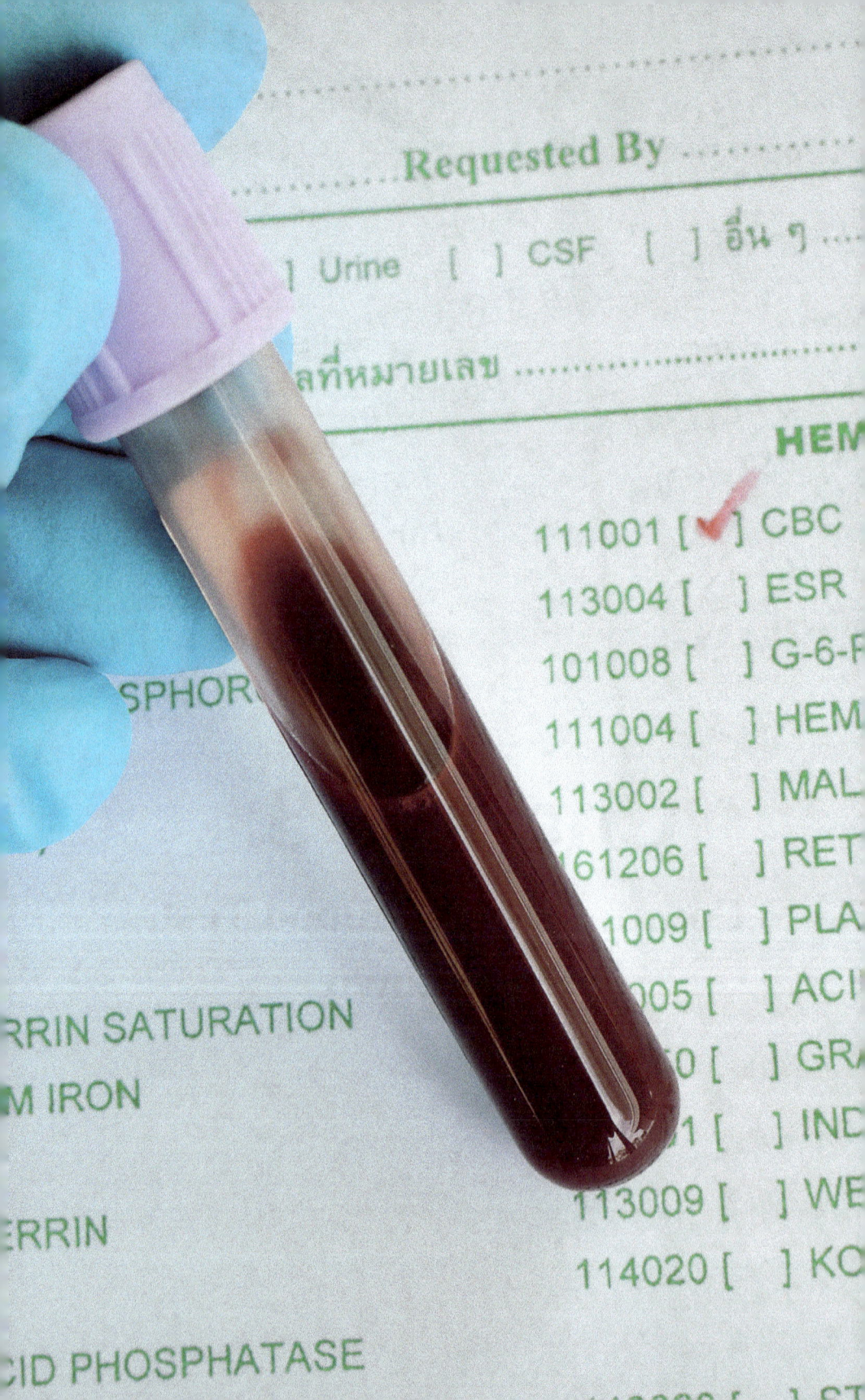

Complete Blood Count (CBC)

In the world of medicine, one of the most common tests performed on patients is a Complete Blood Count (CBC). This test provides valuable information about the different types of cells in your blood and can help diagnose a wide range of conditions, from infections to anemia.

A CBC typically measures three main components of your blood: red blood cells, white blood cells, and platelets. Red blood cells are responsible for carrying oxygen throughout your body, white blood cells help fight off infections, and platelets aid in blood clotting. By analyzing the levels of these cells, healthcare providers can gain insight into your overall health.

When looking at the results of a CBC, it's important to pay attention to a few key indicators. The hemoglobin level, which measures the amount of oxygen-carrying protein in your blood, can indicate if you are anemic. The white blood cell count can show if you have an infection or inflammation in your body. And the platelet count can help identify potential bleeding disorders.

Understanding your CBC results can empower you to take control of your health and work with your healthcare provider to address any potential issues. If you have concerns about your CBC results, don't hesitate to ask your doctor for more information. They can help explain what the results mean and guide you on the best course of action.

By learning more about your Complete Blood Count, you can become a more informed patient and advocate for your own well-being. Remember, knowledge is power when it comes to understanding your medical blood tests.

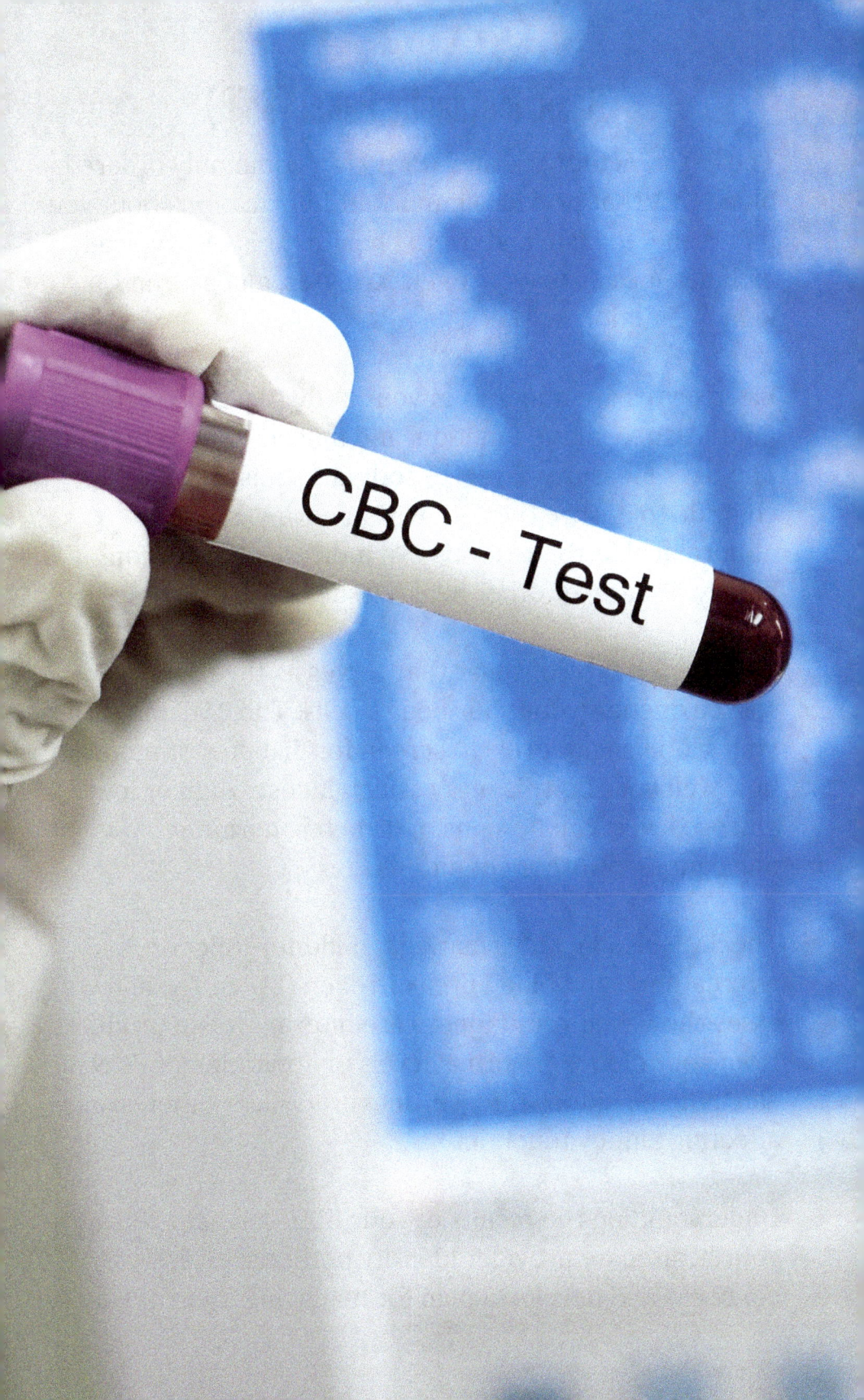

Basic Metabolic Panel (BMP)

The Basic Metabolic Panel (BMP) is a commonly ordered blood test that provides important information about your body's metabolism and overall health. This test typically includes measurements of electrolytes, glucose, and kidney function markers.

Electrolytes are minerals in your body that help regulate fluid balance, nerve function, and muscle contractions. The BMP measures levels of sodium, potassium, and chloride to ensure they are within normal ranges. Abnormal electrolyte levels can indicate dehydration, kidney disease, or other health issues.

Glucose is a type of sugar that serves as the primary source of energy for your body's cells. The BMP measures your blood sugar levels to screen for diabetes or monitor how well your body is processing glucose. High or low glucose levels can be signs of diabetes, hormonal imbalances, or other conditions.

The BMP also includes markers of kidney function, such as creatinine and blood urea nitrogen (BUN). These tests assess how well your kidneys are filtering waste products from your blood. Abnormal levels of creatinine or BUN can indicate kidney disease, dehydration, or other issues affecting kidney function.

Understanding the results of your BMP can help you and your healthcare provider identify potential health concerns and develop a plan for managing them. If you have abnormal results, your doctor may recommend further testing or lifestyle changes to improve your overall health.

By learning more about the Basic Metabolic Panel and how it can provide valuable insights into your health, you can take a proactive approach to monitoring and maintaining your well-being. Remember to discuss your test results with your healthcare provider to ensure you receive appropriate care and support.

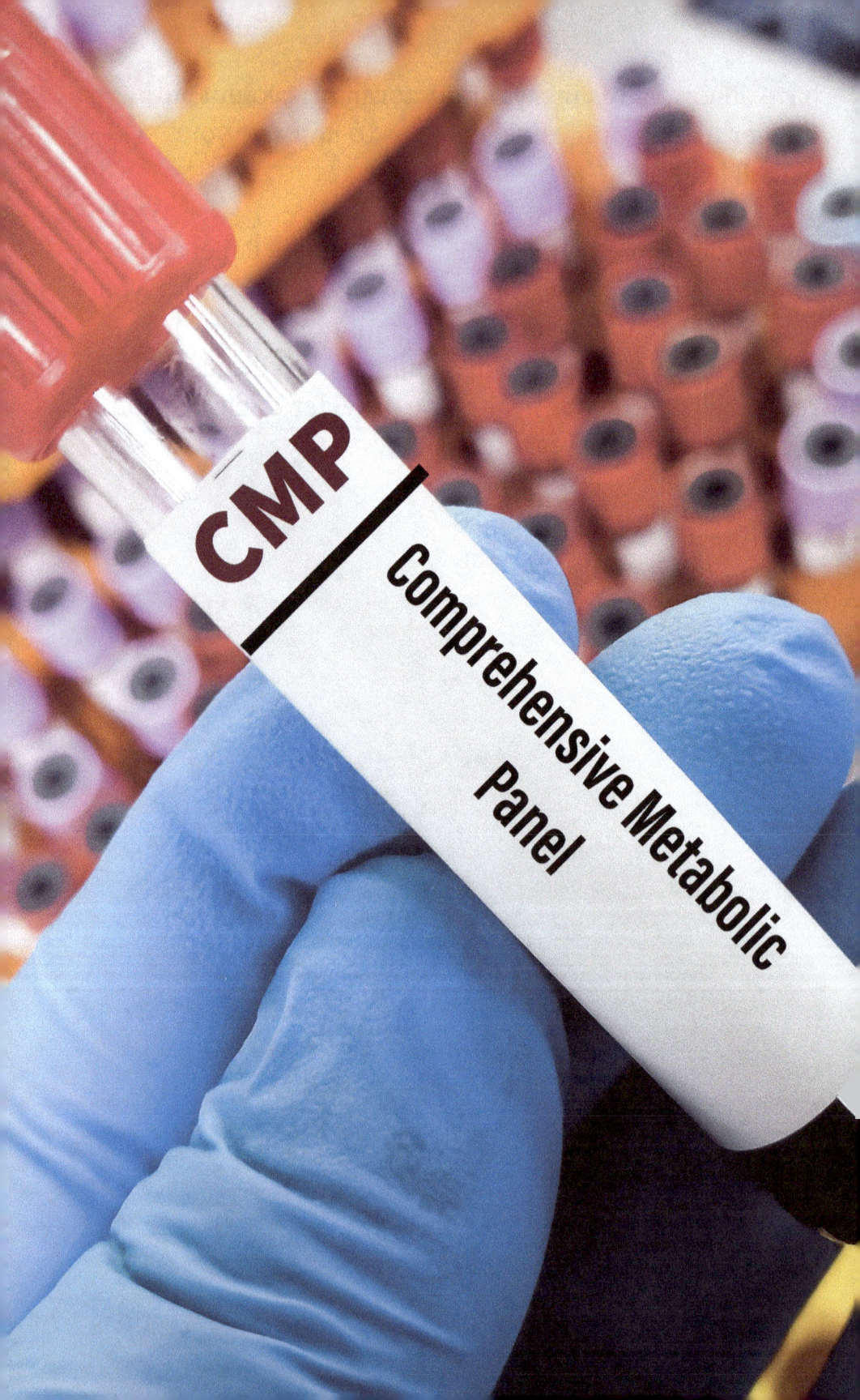

Lipid Panel

A lipid panel is a common blood test that measures the levels of various types of fats in your blood. This test is important because high levels of certain fats, such as cholesterol and triglycerides, can increase your risk of heart disease and other health problems. Understanding your lipid panel results can help you take steps to improve your overall health and reduce your risk of these conditions.

The lipid panel typically includes measurements of total cholesterol, LDL (low-density lipoprotein) cholesterol, HDL (high-density lipoprotein) cholesterol, and triglycerides. Total cholesterol is a combination of LDL and HDL cholesterol, and high levels of total cholesterol can indicate an increased risk of heart disease. LDL cholesterol is often referred to as "bad" cholesterol because high levels can lead to plaque buildup in the arteries. HDL cholesterol, on the other hand, is considered "good" cholesterol because it helps remove LDL cholesterol from the bloodstream.

Triglycerides are another type of fat found in the blood, and high levels can also increase your risk of heart disease. In general, it's important to have a healthy balance of these different types of fats in your blood to maintain good cardiovascular health.

If your lipid panel results show high levels of total cholesterol, LDL cholesterol, or triglycerides, your healthcare provider may recommend lifestyle changes, such as a healthy diet, regular exercise, and medication if necessary. Understanding your lipid panel results and discussing them with your healthcare provider can help you make informed decisions about your health and well-being.

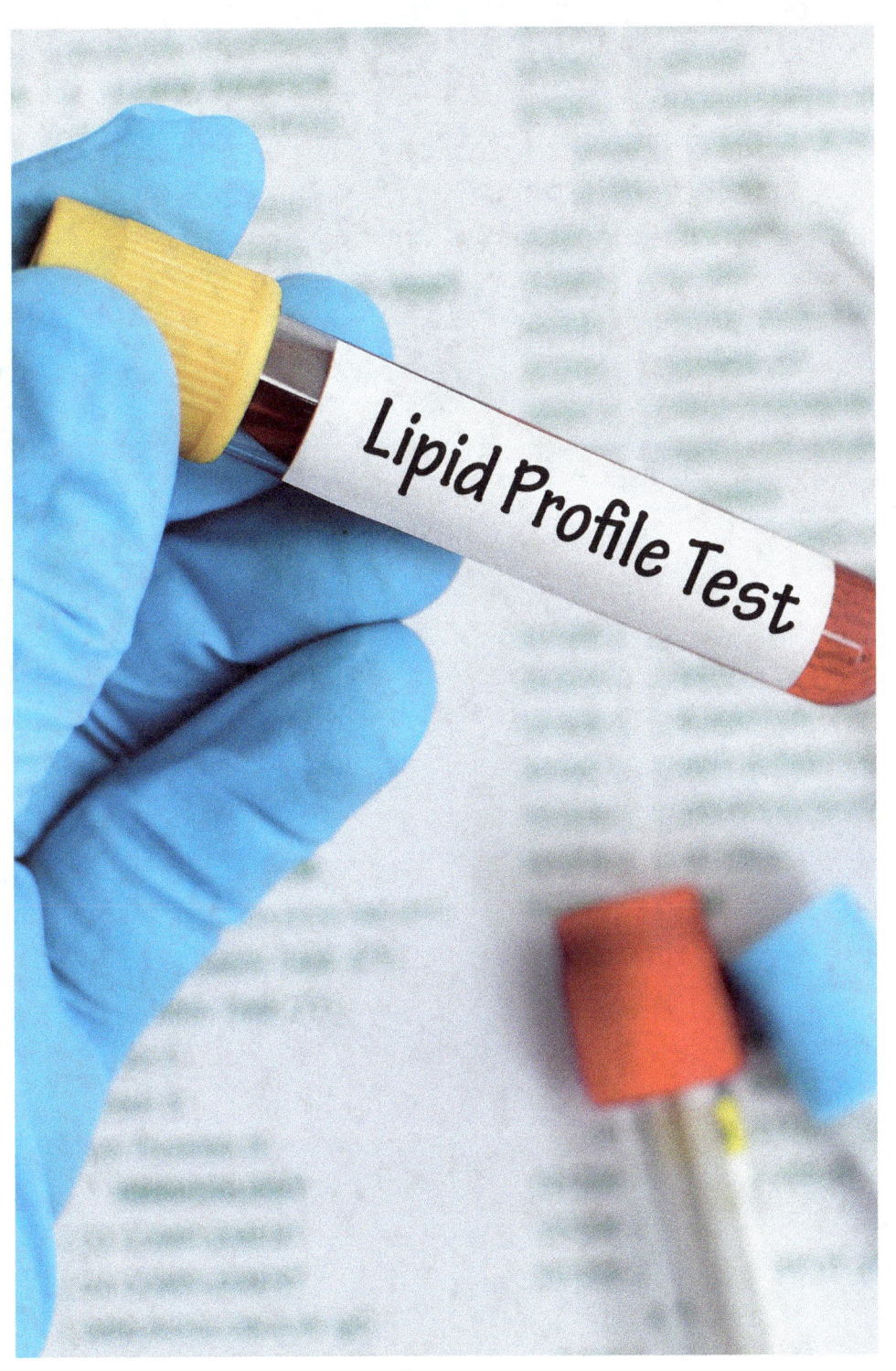

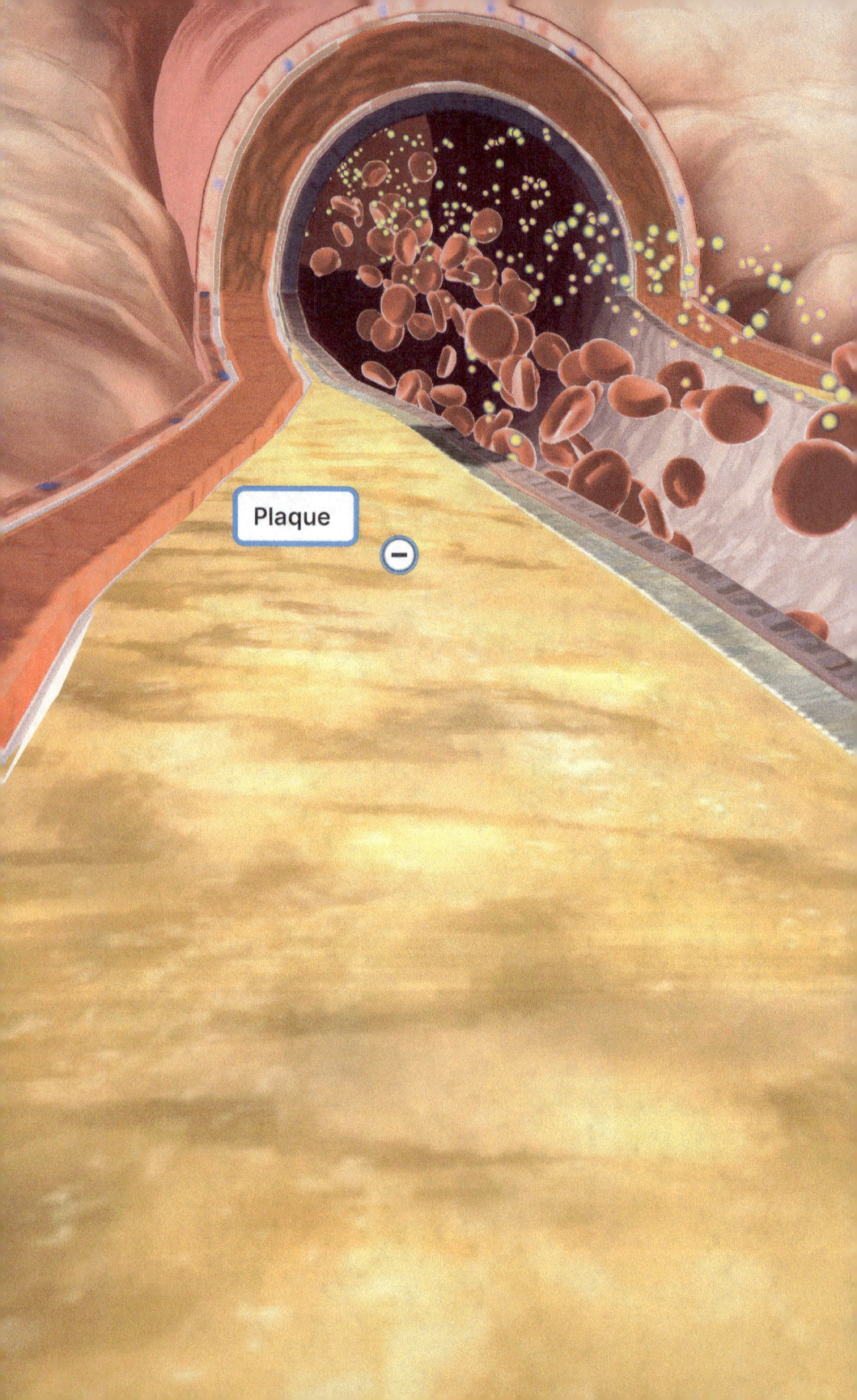

Plaque

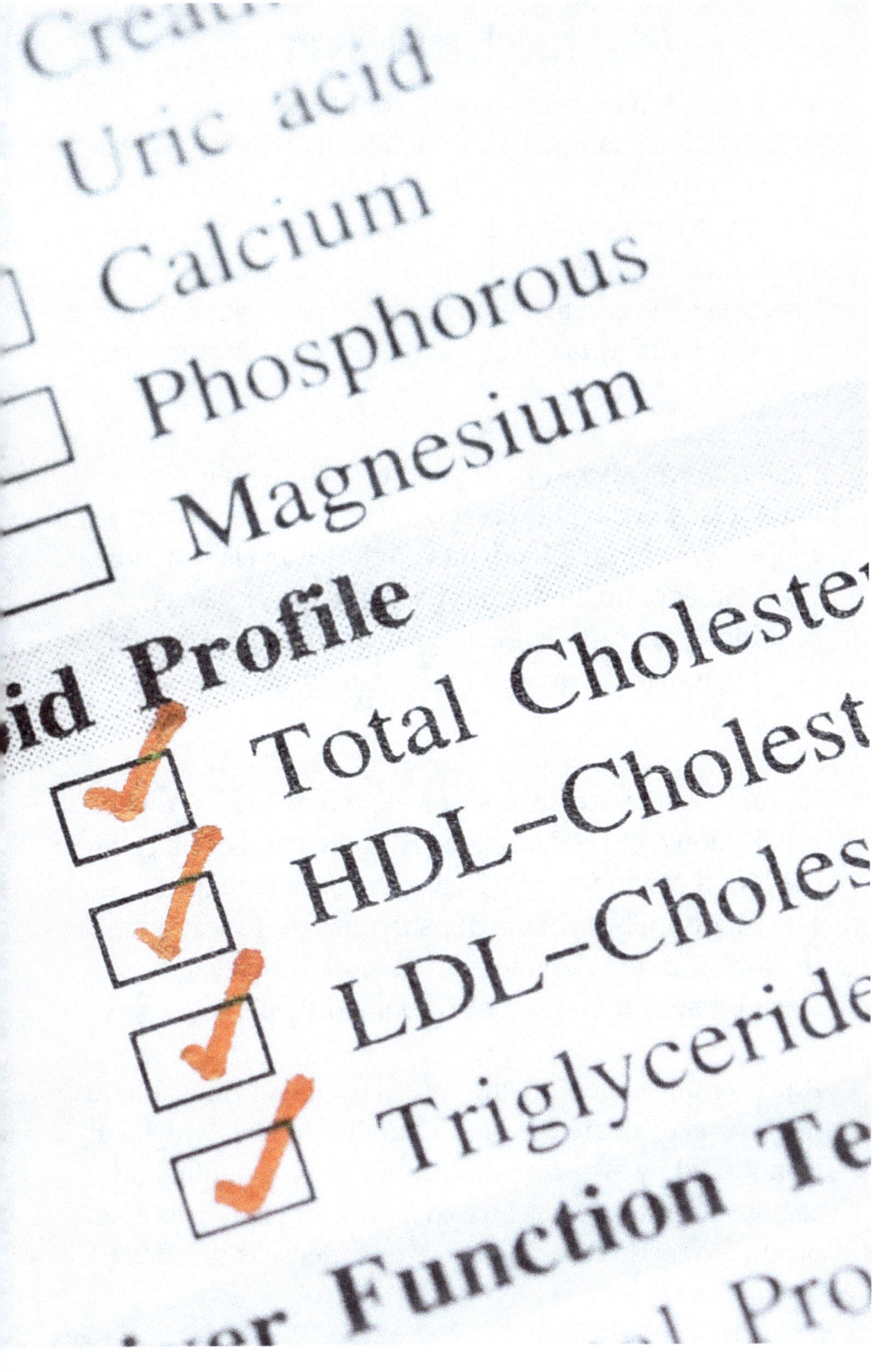

Creat...

Uric acid

Calcium

☐ Phosphorous

☐ Magnesium

id Profile

Total Cholester

☑ HDL-Cholest

☑ LDL-Choles

☑ Triglyceride

er **Function** Te

Pro

Liver Function Tests

Liver function tests are a group of blood tests that provide valuable information about the health of your liver. The liver is a vital organ responsible for processing nutrients, filtering toxins, and producing proteins that are essential for bodily functions. Understanding the results of liver function tests can help you and your healthcare provider assess the function of your liver and identify any potential issues.

One of the key liver function tests is the alanine aminotransferase (ALT) test, which measures the levels of this enzyme in the blood. Elevated ALT levels can indicate liver damage, such as hepatitis or fatty liver disease. Another important test is the aspartate aminotransferase (AST) test, which can also indicate liver damage when elevated.

Bilirubin is a waste product produced by the liver when it breaks down old red blood cells. High levels of bilirubin in the blood can indicate liver disease or bile duct obstruction. The alkaline phosphatase (ALP) test measures the levels of this enzyme in the blood, which can be elevated in liver conditions or bone disorders.

Prothrombin time (PT) and international normalized ratio (INR) tests evaluate the blood's ability to clot, which can be affected by liver disease. Additionally, albumin and total protein tests measure the levels of these proteins produced by the liver, which can be decreased in liver disease.

Understanding the results of liver function tests can help you and your healthcare provider monitor the health of your liver and take appropriate actions if any abnormalities are detected. It is important to discuss your results with your healthcare provider to determine the best course of action for your individual situation.

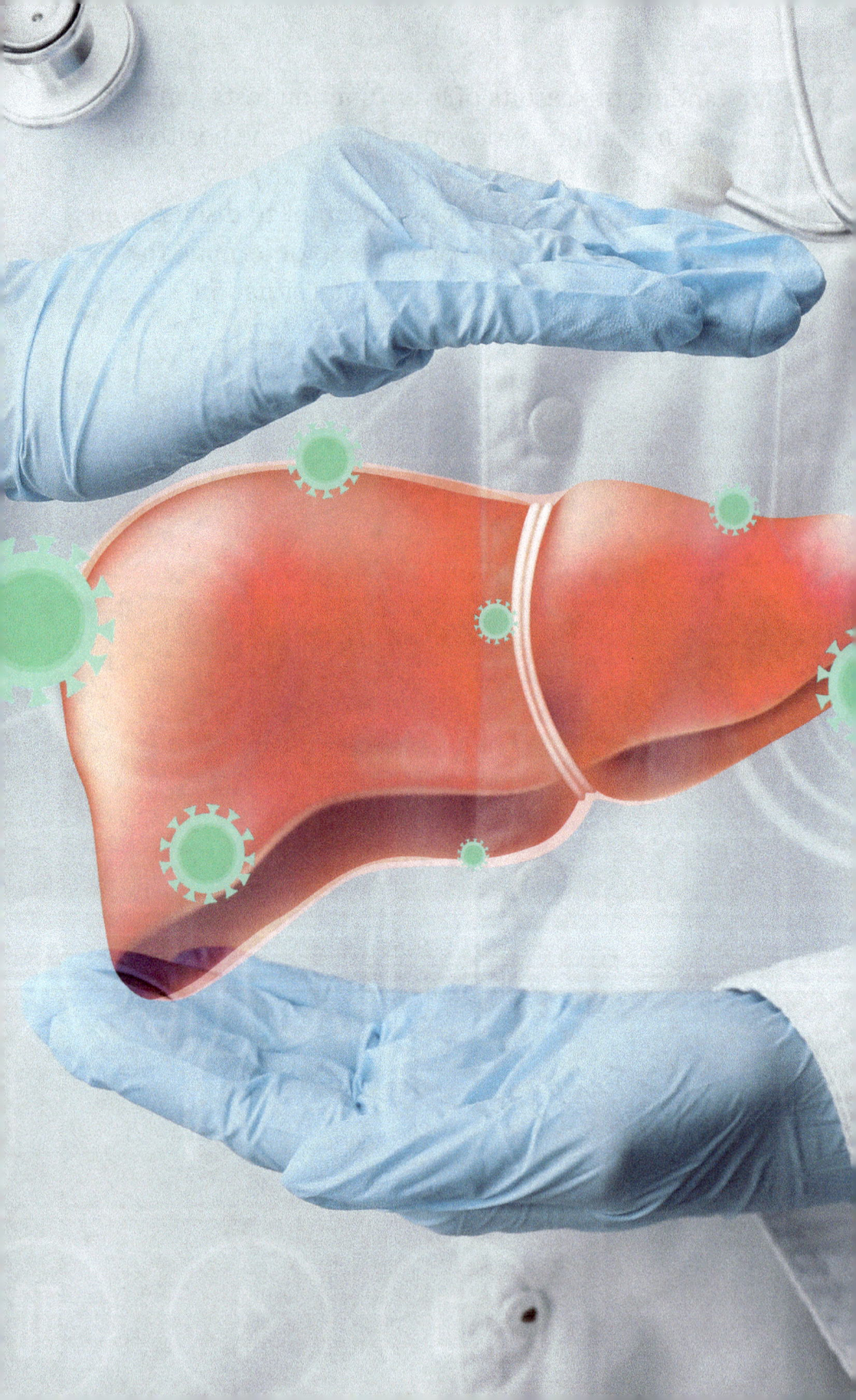

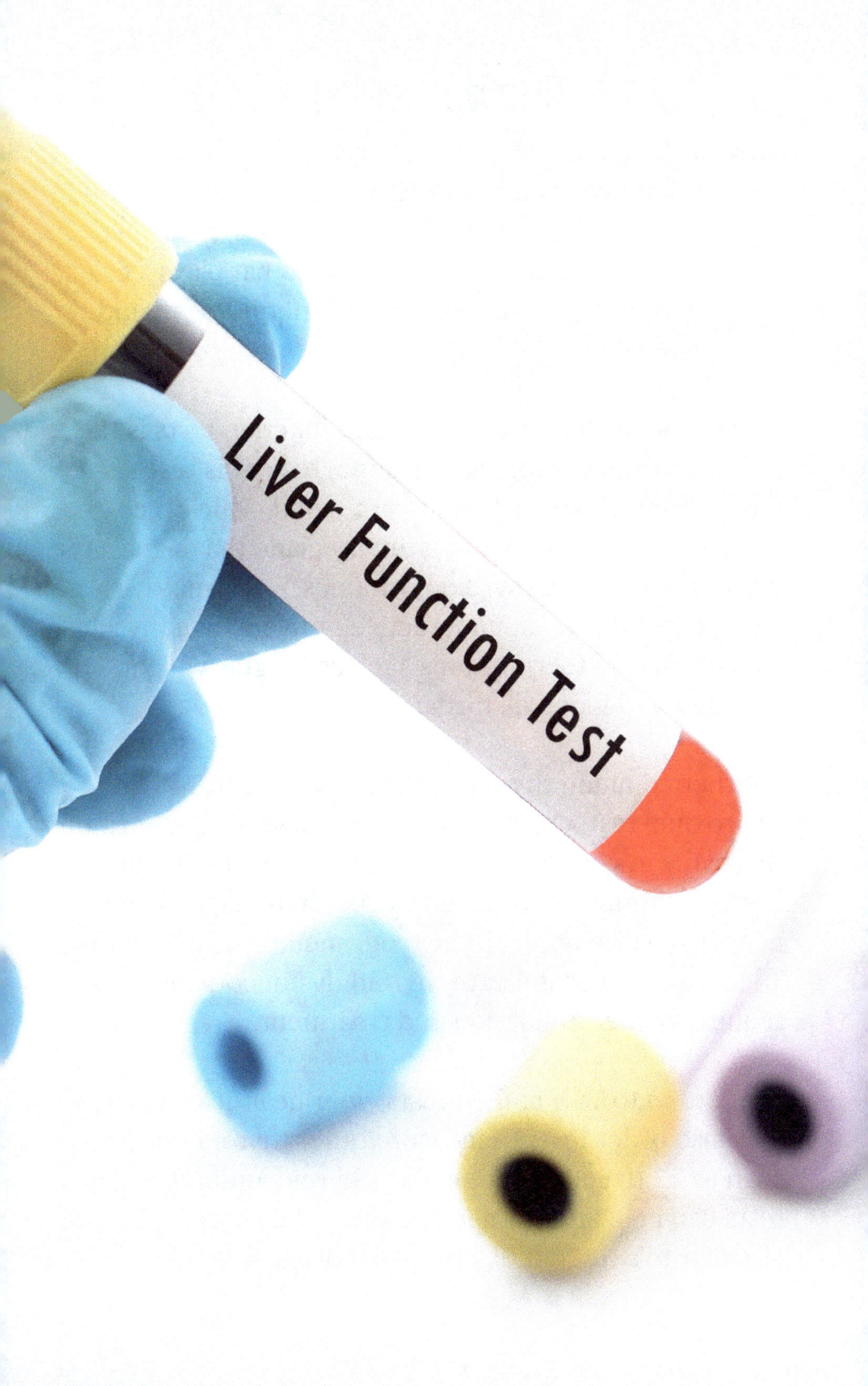

Thyroid Function Tests

Thyroid function tests are a common set of blood tests that can provide valuable insight into the health of your thyroid gland. The thyroid is a small, butterfly-shaped gland located in the front of your neck that plays a crucial role in regulating your metabolism, energy levels, and overall well-being.

One of the most important thyroid function tests is the TSH (thyroid-stimulating hormone) test. This test measures the level of TSH in your blood, which is a hormone produced by the pituitary gland that signals the thyroid to produce thyroid hormones. Abnormal TSH levels can indicate an underactive or overactive thyroid, which can lead to symptoms such as fatigue, weight changes, and mood disturbances.

Another common thyroid function test is the T4 (thyroxine) test, which measures the level of the hormone thyroxine in your blood. Thyroxine is one of the main thyroid hormones produced by the thyroid gland and plays a key role in regulating your metabolism. Abnormal T4 levels can also indicate thyroid dysfunction and may require further evaluation and treatment.

In addition to TSH and T4 tests, your healthcare provider may also order tests to measure other thyroid hormones such as T3 (triiodothyronine) or thyroid antibodies. These tests can help identify specific thyroid disorders such as Hashimoto's thyroiditis or Graves' disease.

Liver Function

Test	
Total Protein	g/L
Albumin	g/L
Globulin	g/L
Total Bilirubin	umol/L
Conjugated Bilirubin	umol/L
Alk.Phosphatase	IU/L
ALT	IU/L
AST	IU/
Gamma GT	IU/

Understanding the results of your thyroid function tests can help you and your healthcare provider determine the best course of action for managing any thyroid issues. By staying informed and proactive about your thyroid health, you can take control of your well-being and make informed decisions about your medical care.

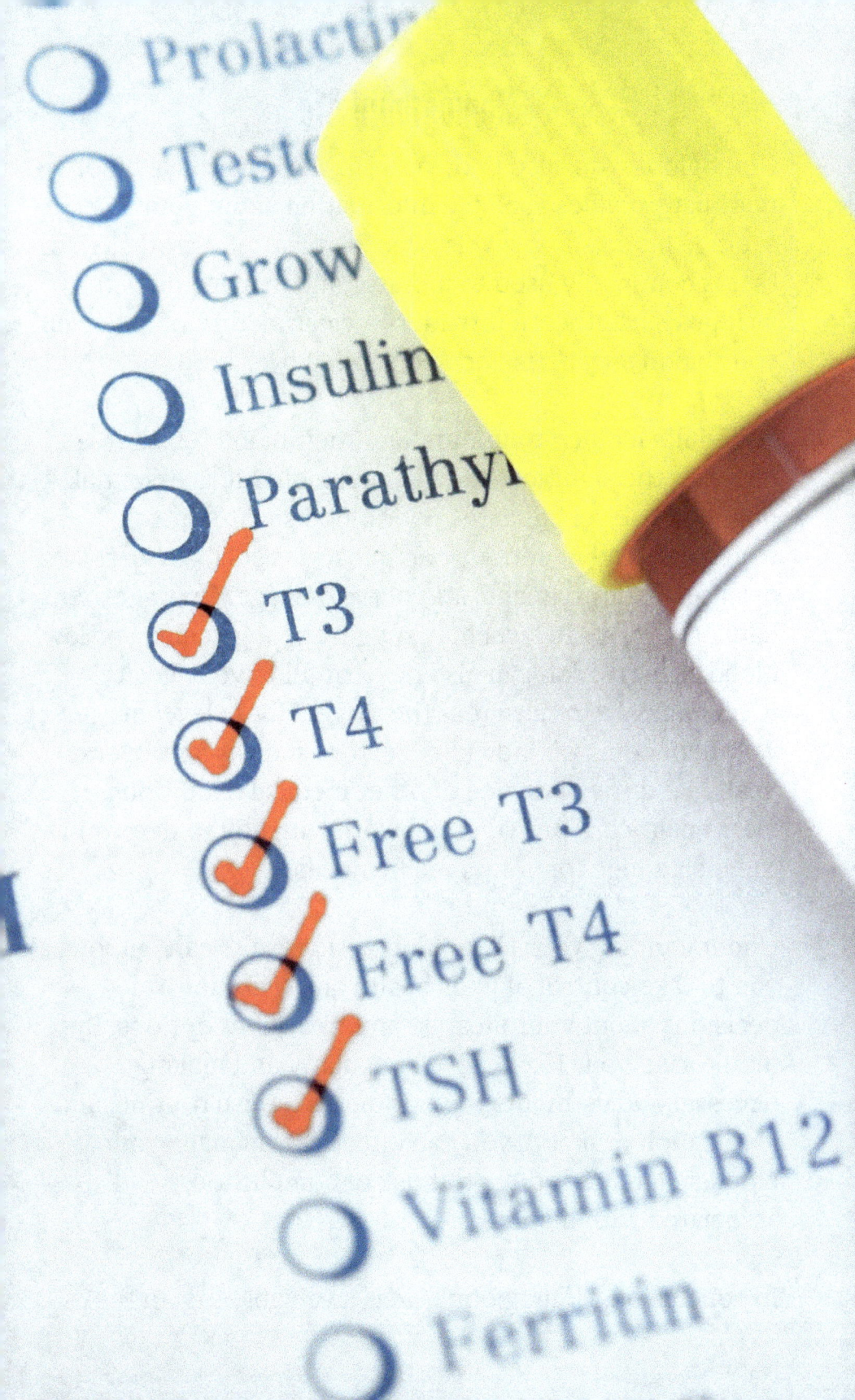

Hemoglobin A1c

Hemoglobin A1c, also known as HbA1c, is a crucial blood test that provides valuable information about your average blood sugar levels over the past 2-3 months. This test is commonly used to monitor and manage diabetes, as it gives healthcare providers a clear picture of how well your blood sugar has been controlled over time.

For adults looking to understand their blood tests, knowing the significance of Hemoglobin A1c is essential. A high HbA1c level indicates poor blood sugar control, which can lead to serious complications such as heart disease, kidney damage, and nerve damage. On the other hand, a low HbA1c level may suggest hypoglycemia, or low blood sugar, which can also be harmful to your health. It is important to note that the target HbA1c level may vary depending on individual factors such as age, overall health, and the presence of other medical conditions. Your healthcare provider will work with you to determine the ideal range for your specific needs.

Understanding your Hemoglobin A1c results can empower you to take control of your health and make informed decisions about your lifestyle and treatment options. By monitoring your HbA1c levels regularly and making necessary adjustments to your diet, exercise routine, and medication regimen, you can effectively manage your blood sugar and reduce the risk of complications associated with diabetes.

In conclusion, Hemoglobin A1c is a valuable tool in the

management of diabetes and provides valuable insights into your overall health. By staying informed and proactive about your blood test results, you can work towards achieving optimal health and well-being.

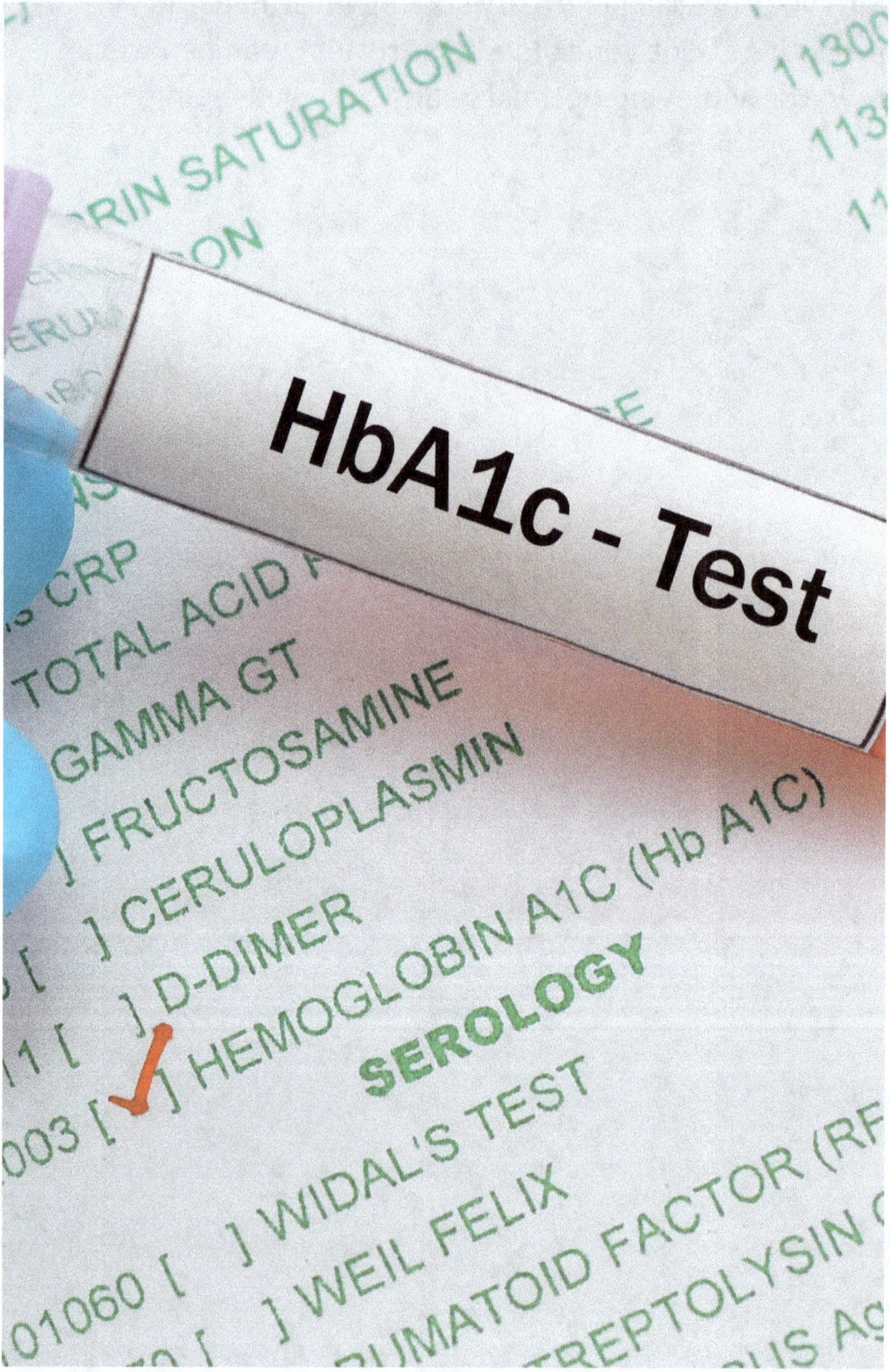
HbA1c - Test
RIN SATURATION
TOTAL ACID
GAMMA GT
] FRUCTOSAMINE
] CERULOPLASMIN
] D-DIMER
003 [ ] HEMOGLOBIN A1C (Hb A1C)
SEROLOGY
] WIDAL'S TEST
01060 [ ] WEIL FELIX
UMATOID FACTOR (RF
TREPTOLYSIN

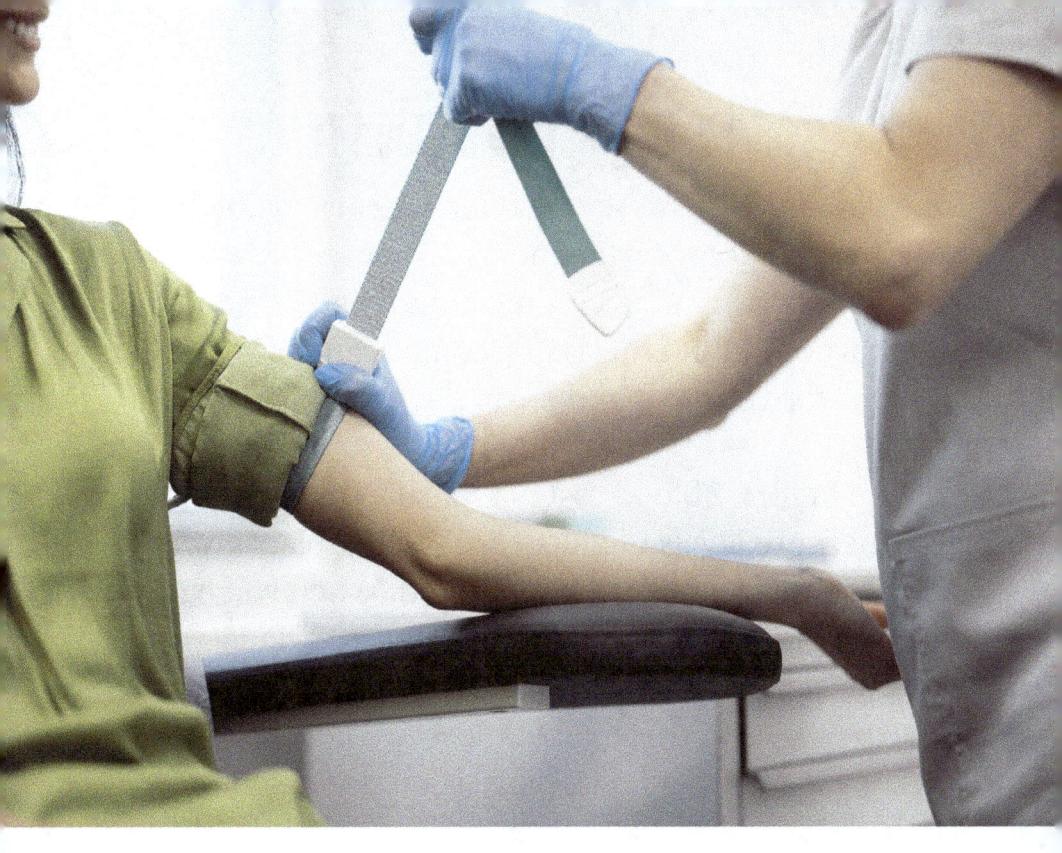

Chapter 4:

Tips for Preparing for a Blood Test

Fasting Before a Blood Test

One common instruction you may receive before a blood test is to fast for a certain period of time. But why is fasting necessary before some blood tests? Understanding the reasons behind this requirement can help you better prepare for your test and ensure accurate results.

Fasting before a blood test is typically required for tests that measure levels of glucose, cholesterol, triglycerides, and certain hormones in your blood. When you eat, your body metabolizes the food and releases various substances into your bloodstream. Fasting helps to ensure that the levels of these substances are not influenced by recent meals, providing a more accurate baseline for comparison.

For example, fasting before a cholesterol test helps to measure your fasting lipid profile, which provides a clearer picture of your cholesterol levels. If you eat before the test, your triglyceride levels may be temporarily elevated, leading to inaccurate results.

It is usually recommended to fast for at least 8-12 hours before a blood test, although the specific fasting requirements may vary depending on the test being performed. During this fasting period, you should avoid consuming anything other than water. Certain medications may also need to be avoided or taken with caution during fasting, so be sure to follow your healthcare provider's instructions carefully.

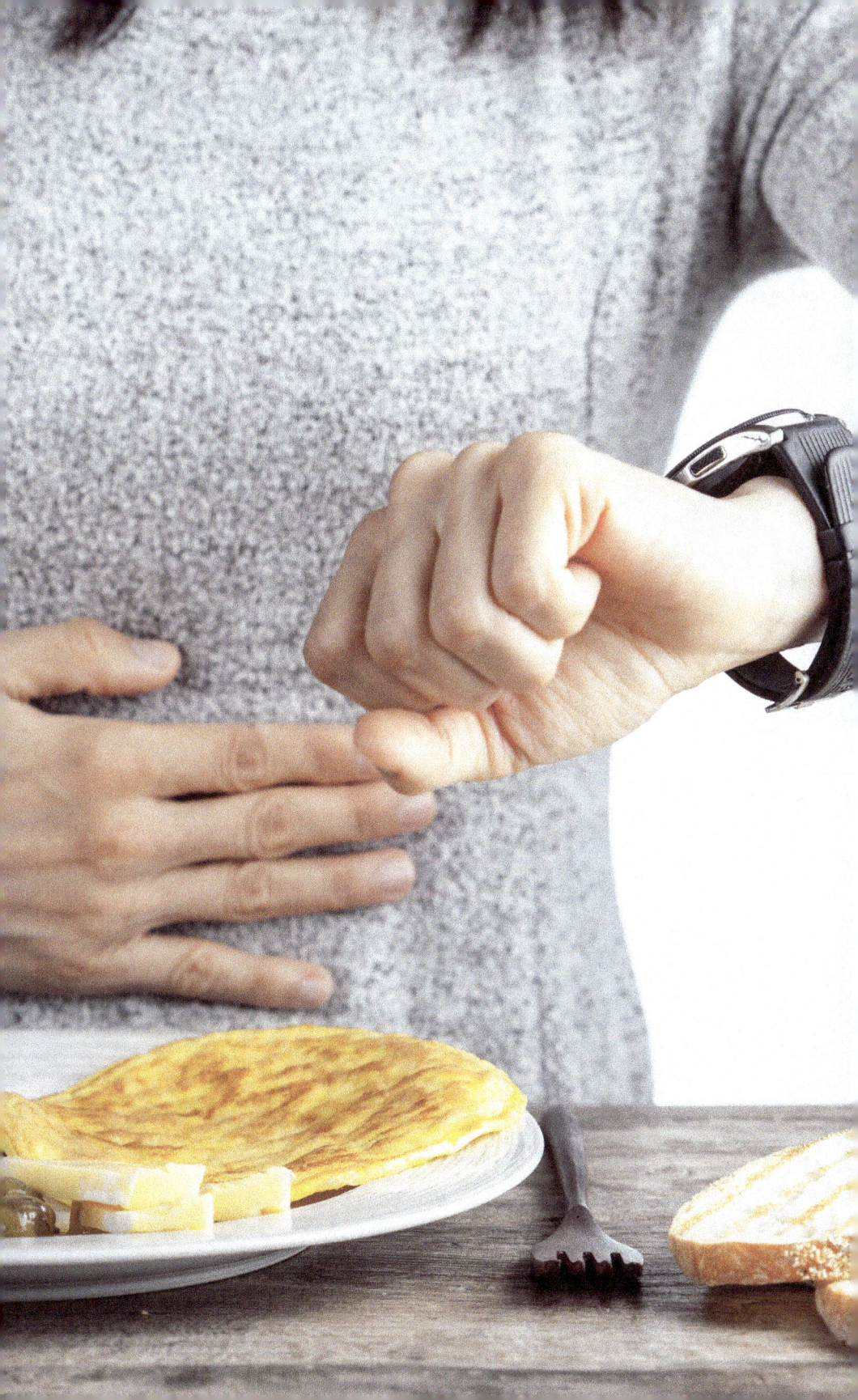

By following the fasting guidelines provided before your blood test, you can help ensure that your results are accurate and reliable. Understanding the importance of fasting before certain blood tests can empower you to take an active role in your healthcare and make informed decisions based on your test results.

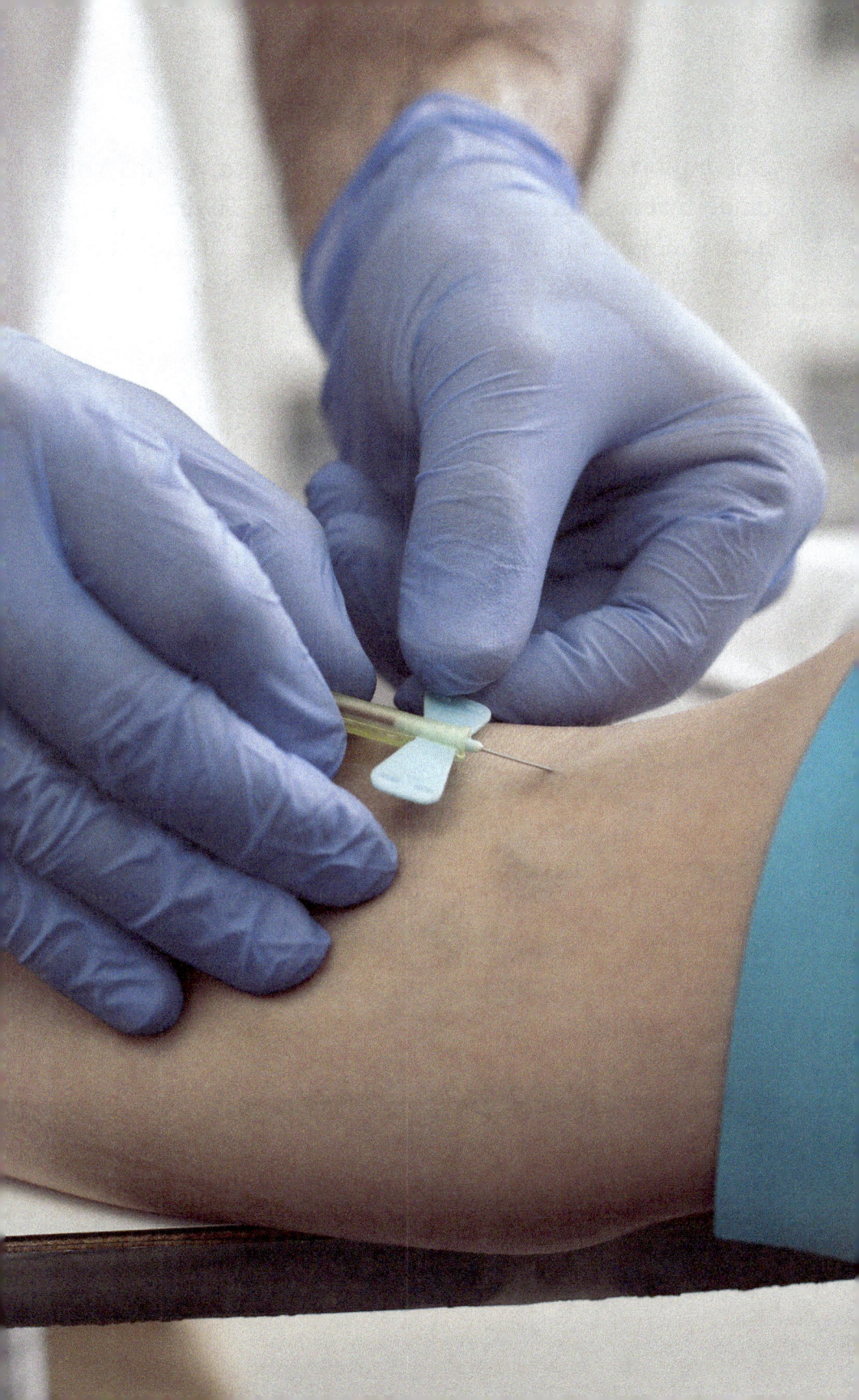

Hydration and Blood Tests

One important factor to consider when interpreting your blood test results is your hydration levels. Hydration can have a significant impact on the results of certain blood tests, so it's essential to understand how it can affect your results.

When you are dehydrated, your blood becomes more concentrated, which can affect the levels of various components in your blood. For example, if you are dehydrated, your sodium levels may appear higher than they actually are. On the other hand, if you are overhydrated, your sodium levels may appear lower than they actually are. This is why it's crucial to ensure that you are properly hydrated before undergoing any blood tests.

To ensure accurate results, it is recommended to drink plenty of water in the hours leading up to your blood test. However, it is also important not to overhydrate, as this can also affect your results. It's best to follow your healthcare provider's instructions regarding fasting and hydration before your blood test to ensure the most accurate results.

It's important to note that certain blood tests, such as those measuring electrolyte levels, may require specific instructions regarding hydration and fasting. It's essential to follow these instructions carefully to ensure accurate results.

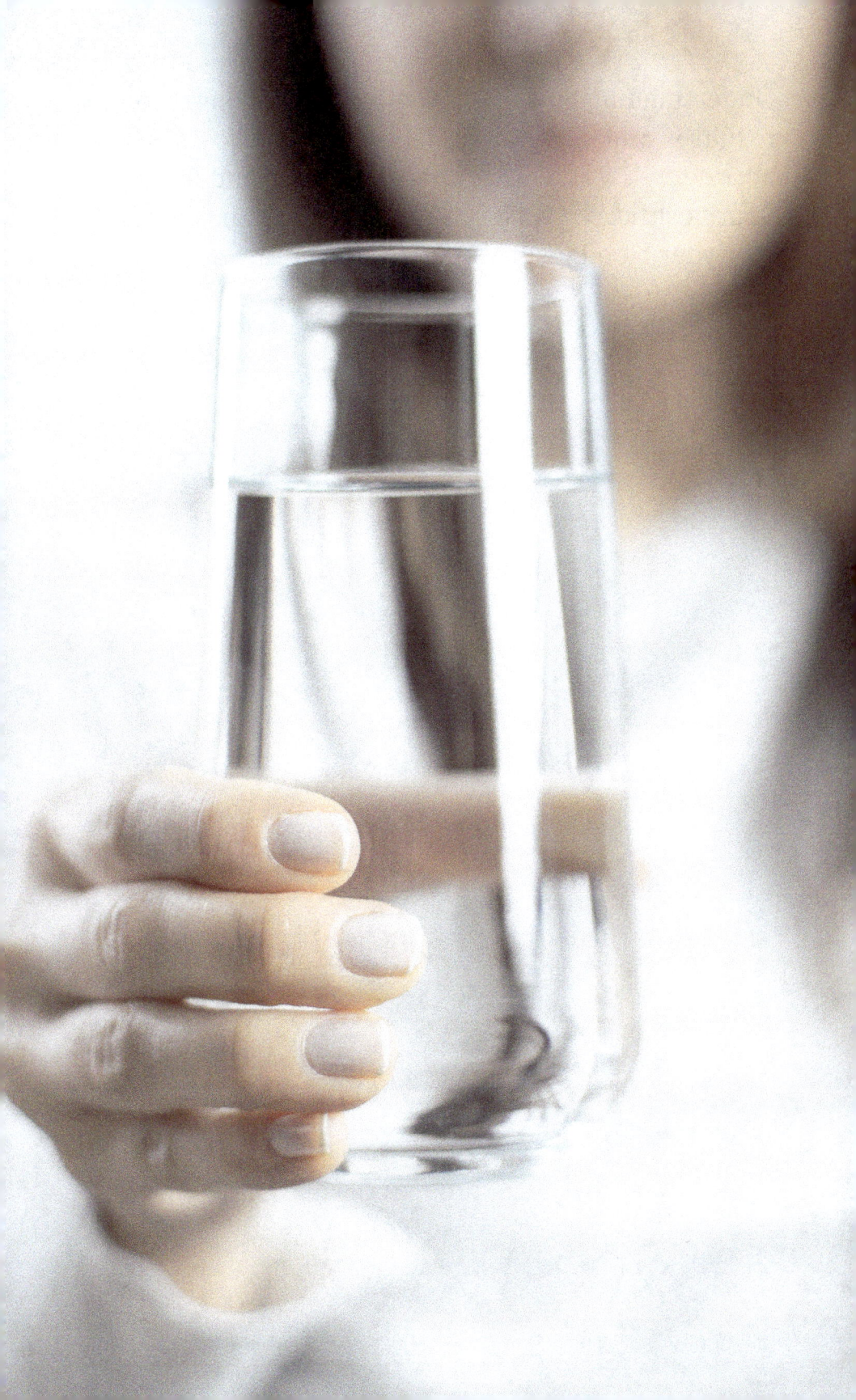

Understanding how hydration can affect your blood test results is crucial for interpreting your medical results accurately. By staying properly hydrated and following your healthcare provider's instructions, you can ensure that your blood test results are as accurate as possible.

Medications and Blood Test Results

Understanding your blood test results can be overwhelming, especially when it comes to interpreting the impact of medications on your results. Medications can have a significant influence on your blood test outcomes, affecting everything from cholesterol levels to blood sugar readings. In this subchapter, we will delve into the relationship between medications and blood test results, providing you with the knowledge you need to make sense of your medical reports.

Certain medications can cause fluctuations in your blood test results, leading to inaccurate readings that may not reflect your true health status. For example, statins, commonly prescribed for high cholesterol, can impact liver function tests, while corticosteroids can affect glucose levels. It is crucial to inform your healthcare provider about all the medications you are taking before undergoing blood tests to ensure that the results are interpreted correctly.

Additionally, understanding how medications interact with each other is essential for managing your health effectively. Some medications can interact negatively with each other, leading to adverse effects on your blood test results. By being aware of potential interactions, you can work with your healthcare provider to adjust your medication regimen and optimize your treatment plan.

By educating yourself about the relationship between medications and blood test results, you can take control

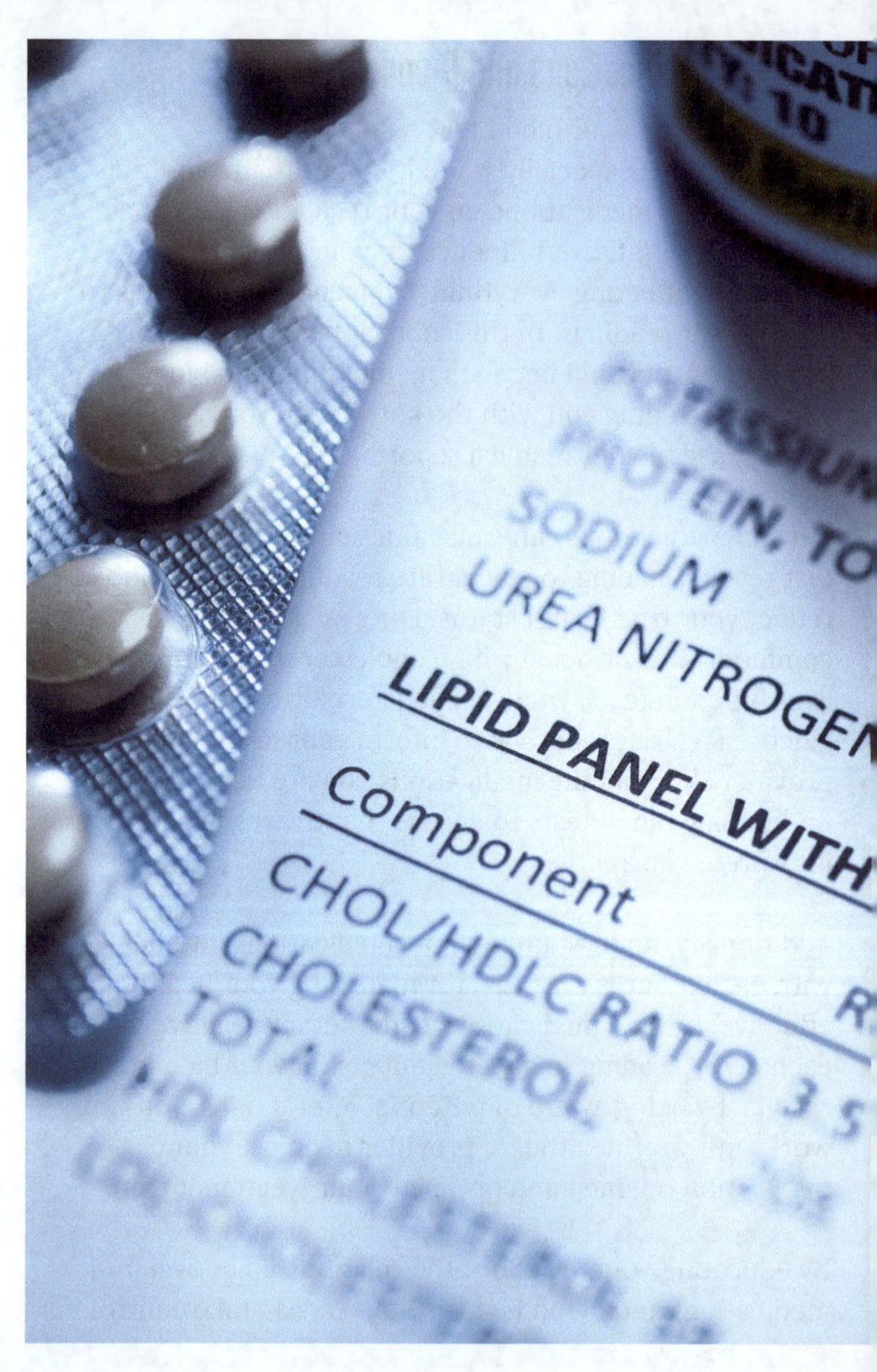

of your health and make informed decisions about your treatment. Armed with this knowledge, you will be better equipped to collaborate with your healthcare provider in interpreting your blood test results accurately and developing a personalized care plan that meets your unique needs.

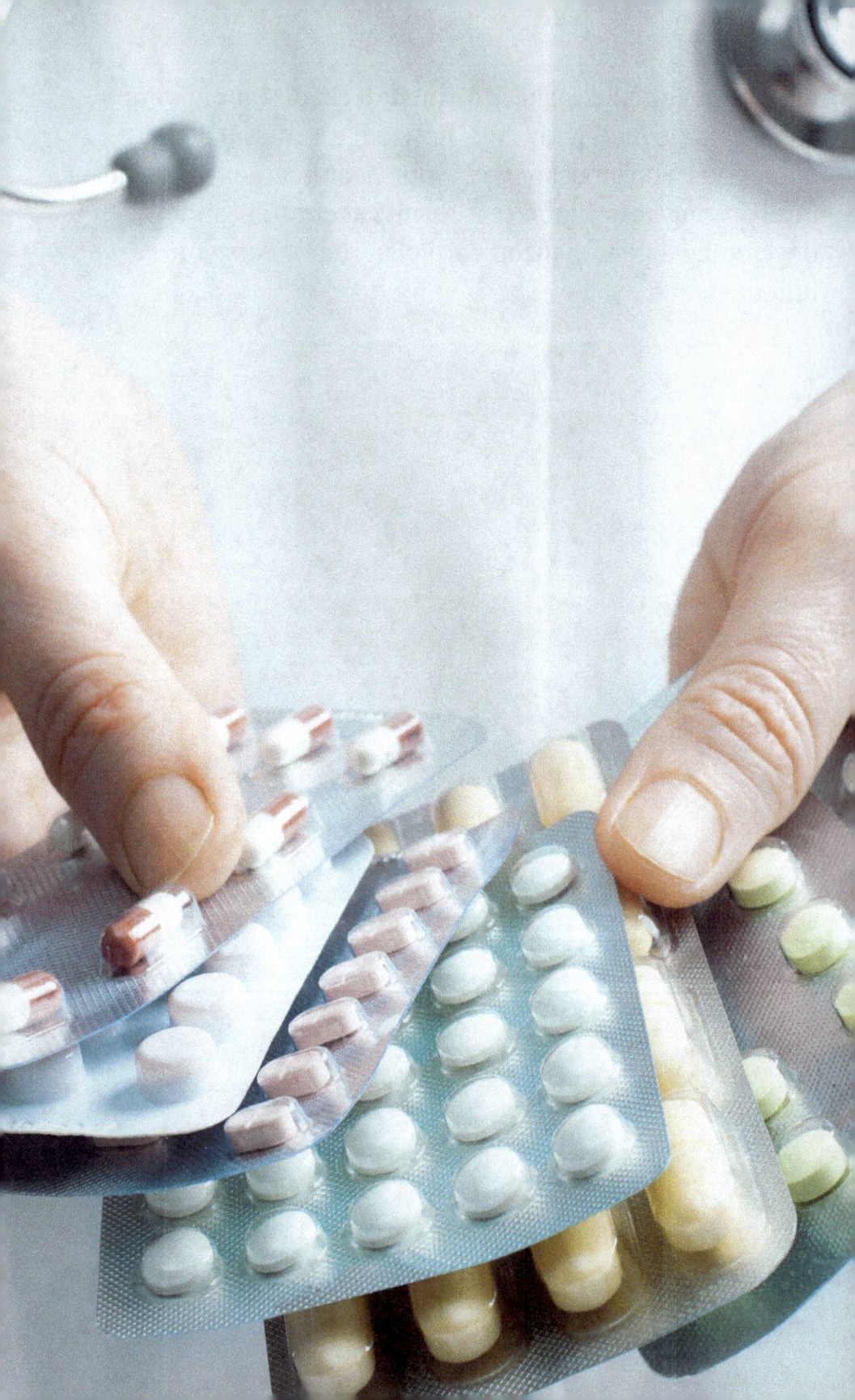

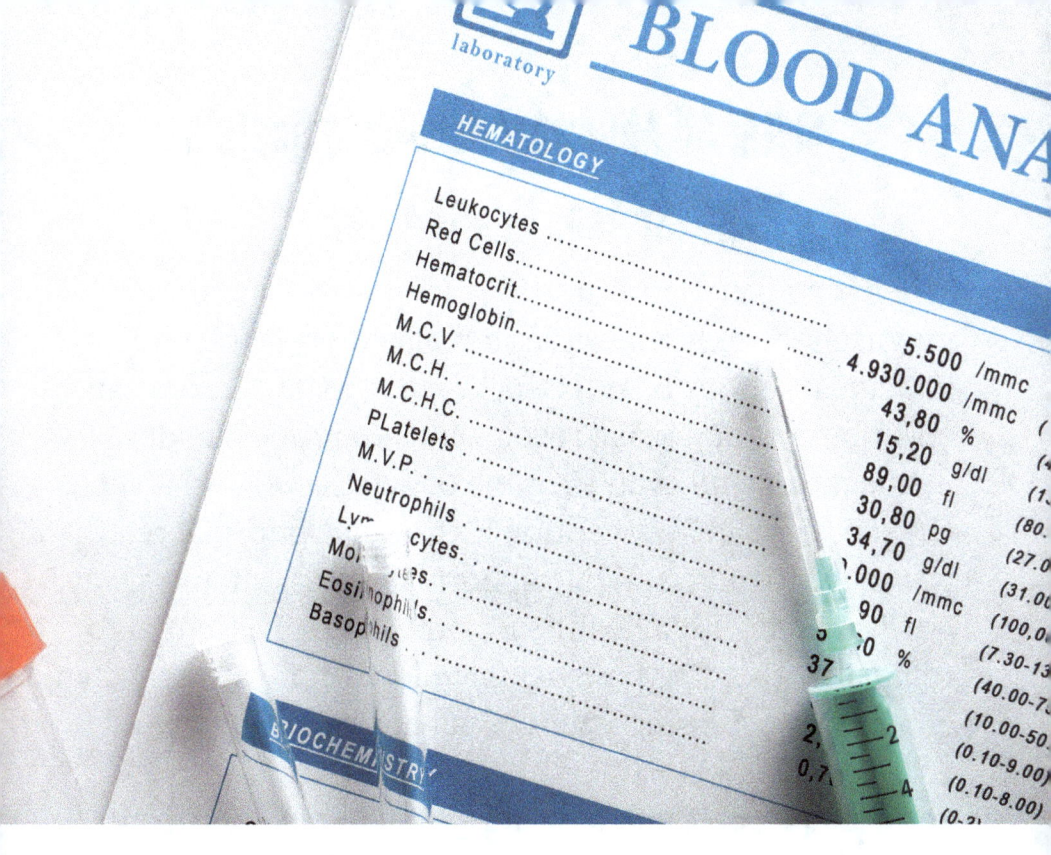

Chapter 5:

Common Misconceptions About Blood Tests

Myth: All Abnormal Results Indicate a Serious Health Issue

When it comes to interpreting blood test results, it's important to remember that not all abnormal results indicate a serious health issue. In fact, many factors can contribute to abnormal results, including age, gender, medications, and even the time of day the test was taken. One common misconception is that any abnormal result is a cause for alarm. While abnormal results should always be discussed with a healthcare provider, it's essential to remember that they are just one piece of the puzzle when it comes to assessing your overall health.

For example, certain medications or supplements can cause fluctuations in blood test results. Additionally, some conditions may cause temporary abnormalities that resolve on their own. By working closely with your healthcare provider, you can better understand the context of your results and determine the appropriate next steps.

It's also important to keep in mind that not all abnormalities are created equal. Some abnormalities may be minor and require no further action, while others may indicate a more serious underlying health issue. Your healthcare provider will be able to help you navigate your results and determine the best course of action.

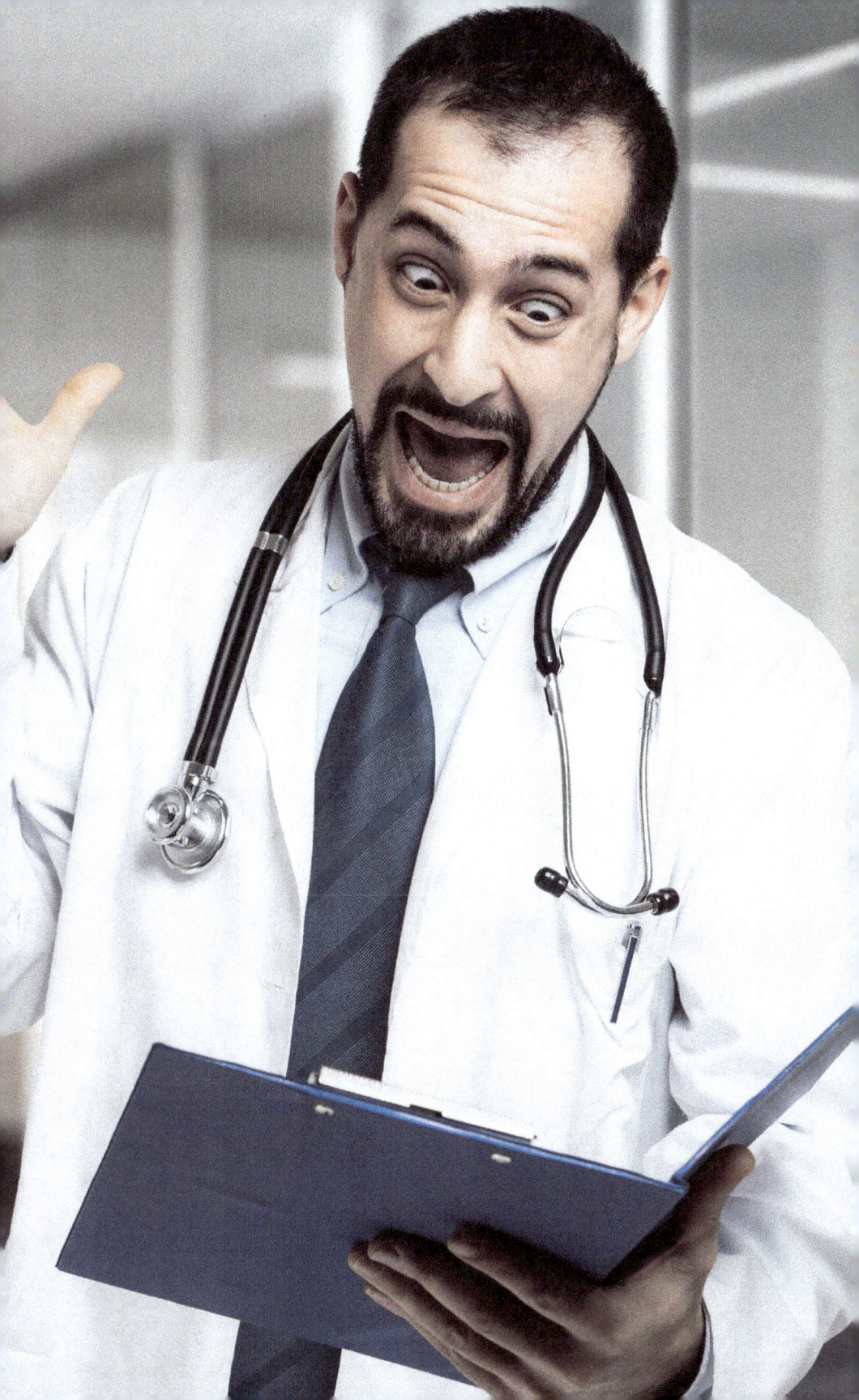

By understanding that not all abnormal results are cause for alarm, you can approach your blood test results with a sense of perspective and empowerment. Remember, knowledge is power when it comes to your health, and being proactive about understanding your results is an essential step in taking control of your well-being.

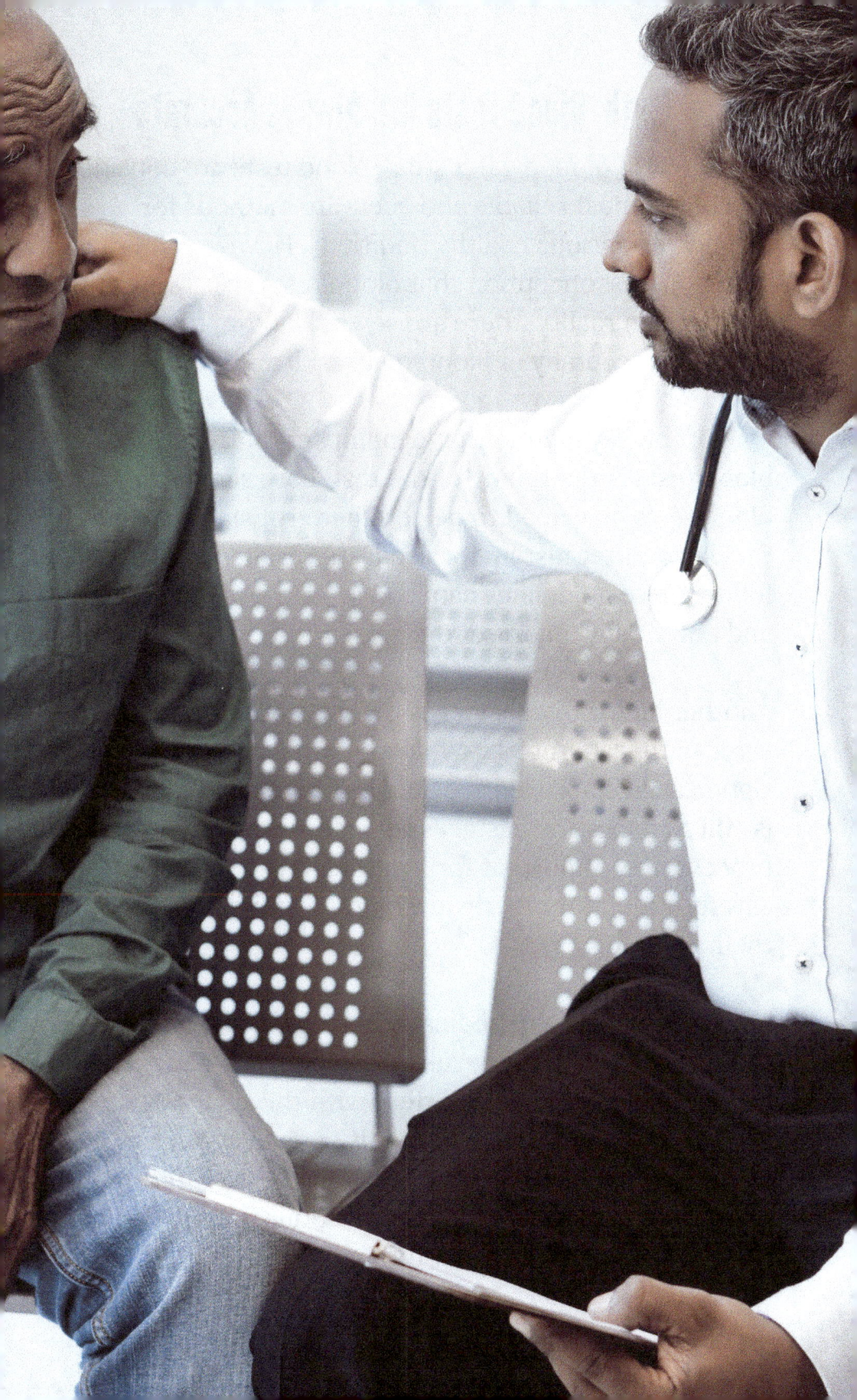

Myth: Blood Tests Are Always Accurate

In the world of medical testing, blood tests are considered one of the most reliable and accurate methods for diagnosing various health conditions. However, it is a common misconception that blood tests are always 100% accurate. In reality, there are several factors that can affect the accuracy of blood test results.

One of the key factors that can impact the accuracy of blood tests is the timing of the test. For example, certain blood tests may need to be conducted at specific times of the day or after fasting for accurate results. Failure to follow these guidelines can lead to inaccurate readings and potentially incorrect diagnoses.

Another factor to consider is the possibility of human error in the laboratory. While modern technology has significantly improved the accuracy of blood tests, there is still a chance for mistakes to occur during the testing process. It is important for healthcare providers to carefully monitor and review blood test results to ensure their accuracy.

Additionally, certain medications or medical conditions can also influence the results of blood tests. For example, some medications can interfere with the accuracy of certain blood tests, leading to false positive or false negative results. It is crucial for individuals to inform their healthcare providers of any medications they are taking or pre-existing medical conditions before undergoing blood tests.

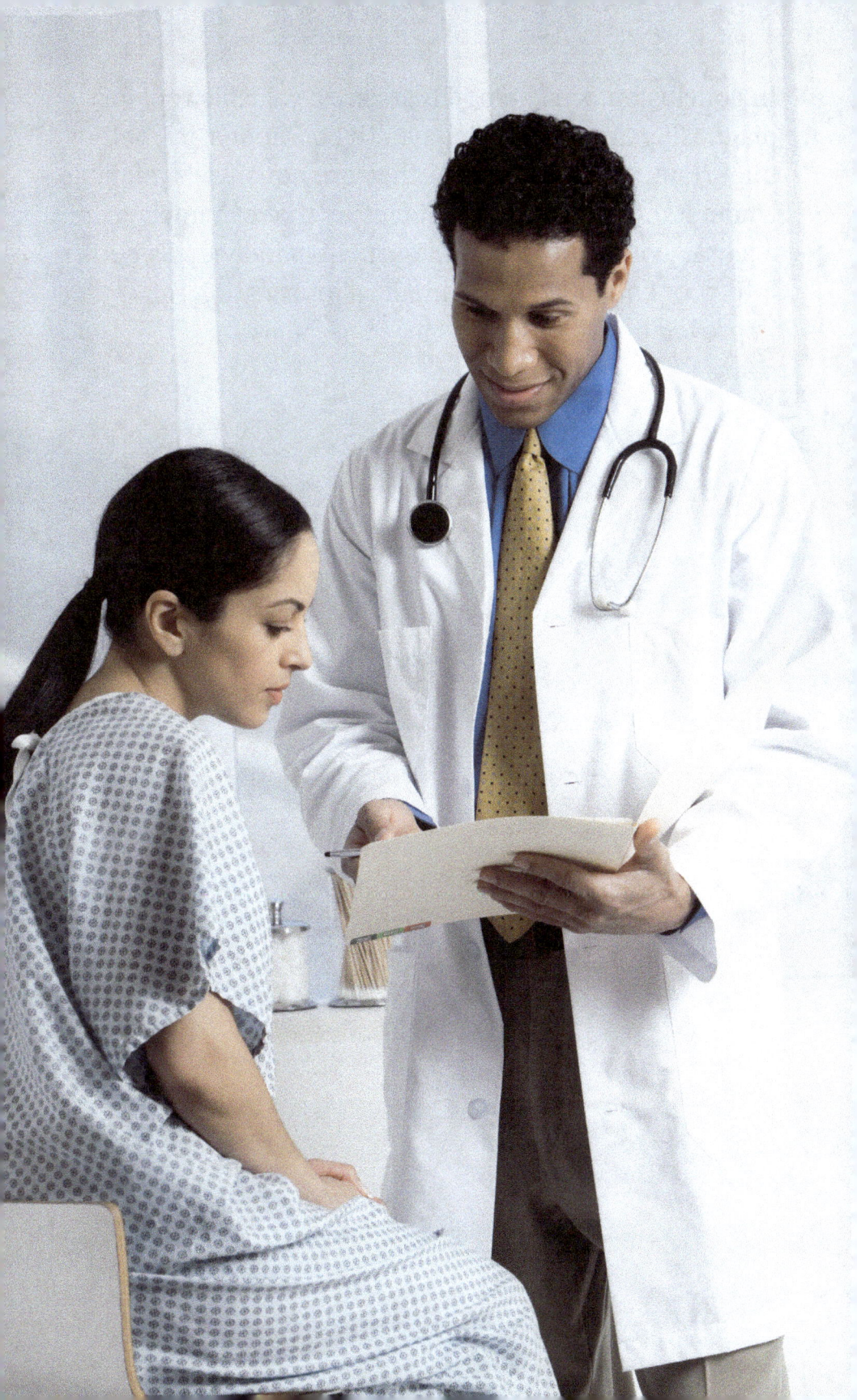

In conclusion, while blood tests are a valuable tool for diagnosing and monitoring health conditions, it is important to recognize that they are not always infallible. Understanding the potential factors that can impact the accuracy of blood test results can help individuals better interpret and utilize their medical information for improved health outcomes.

Myth: You Don't Need to Understand Your Blood Test Results

One common myth surrounding blood test results is that you don't need to understand them in order to benefit from the information they provide. This couldn't be further from the truth. Understanding your blood test results is crucial in order to take control of your health and make informed decisions about your well-being.

When you receive your blood test results, it can be tempting to simply hand them over to your doctor and trust that they will take care of everything. However, by taking the time to understand what the different values and markers mean, you can become an active participant in your own healthcare.

By understanding your blood test results, you can gain valuable insights into your overall health and well-being. You can identify any potential red flags or areas of concern that may require further investigation. This knowledge can empower you to make lifestyle changes, seek out additional testing, or follow up with your healthcare provider to address any issues that may arise.

Additionally, understanding your blood test results can help you track your progress over time. By keeping a record of your results and comparing them to previous tests, you can monitor changes in your health and make adjustments as needed. This can be especially helpful for individuals managing chronic conditions or working

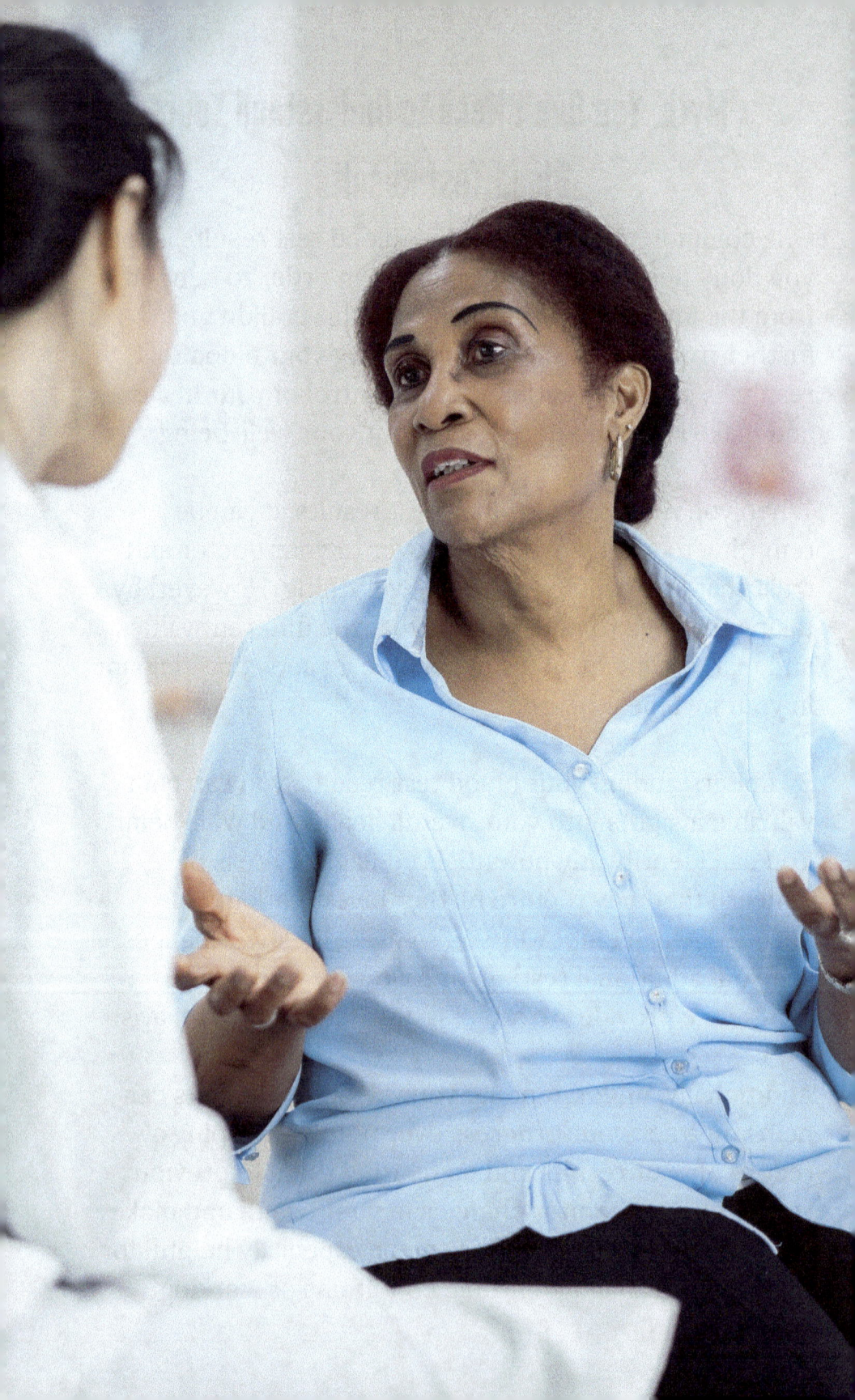

towards specific health goals.

In conclusion, don't fall victim to the myth that you don't need to understand your blood test results. By taking the time to educate yourself and ask questions, you can become a more informed and proactive participant in your healthcare journey. Your blood test results are a valuable tool in helping you achieve optimal health and well-being, so make sure you take the time to understand them.

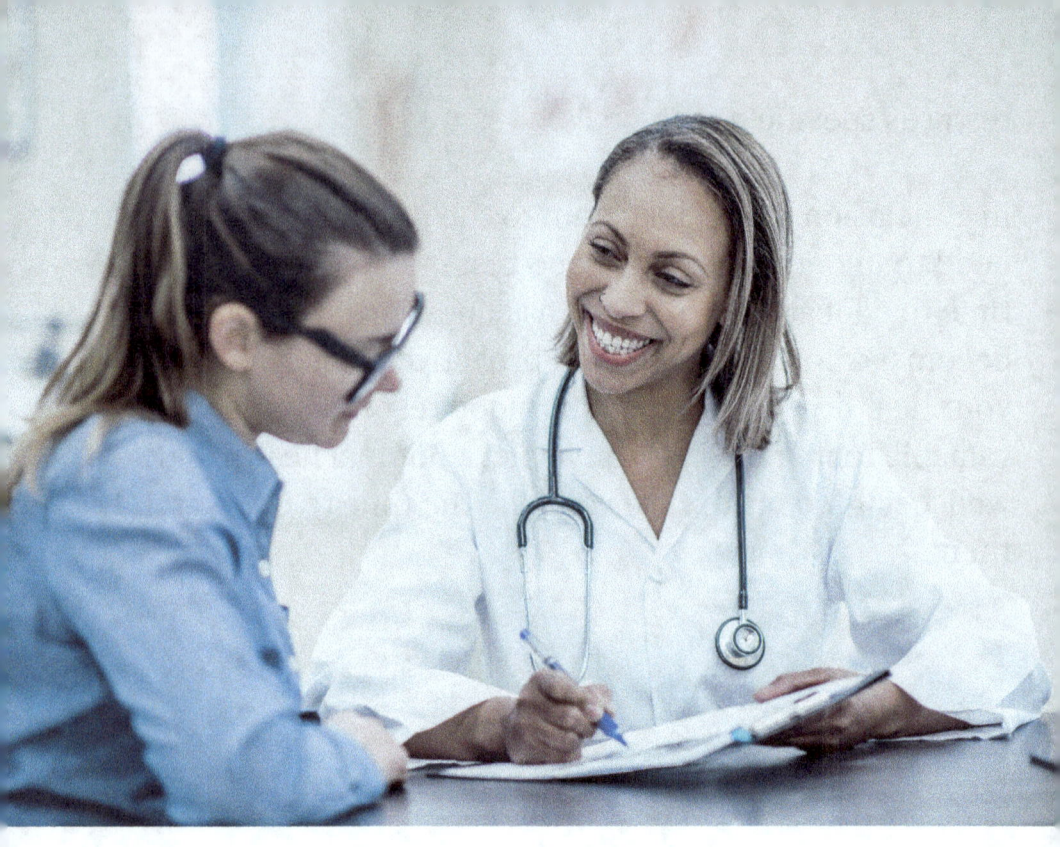

Chapter 6:

Communicating with Your Healthcare Provider About Blood Tests

Questions to Ask Your Doctor About Your Blood Test Results

If you're like most adults, you've probably had blood tests done at some point in your life. And if you're like many people, you may have been left scratching your head when you received the results. Understanding your blood test results can be confusing, but it's important to know what they mean for your health.

When you receive your blood test results from your doctor, don't be afraid to ask questions. Your doctor is there to help you understand your health and make informed decisions about your care. Here are some important questions to ask your doctor about your blood test results:

1. What do my blood test results mean? Your doctor can help you interpret your results and explain what they indicate about your health. They can also let you know if any further testing or treatment is needed.

2. Are my results normal? Your doctor can tell you if your results fall within the normal range for your age and gender, or if they indicate any abnormalities that may require further investigation.

3. What are the possible causes of any abnormal results? Your doctor can help you understand what might be causing any abnormal results and discuss potential treatment options.

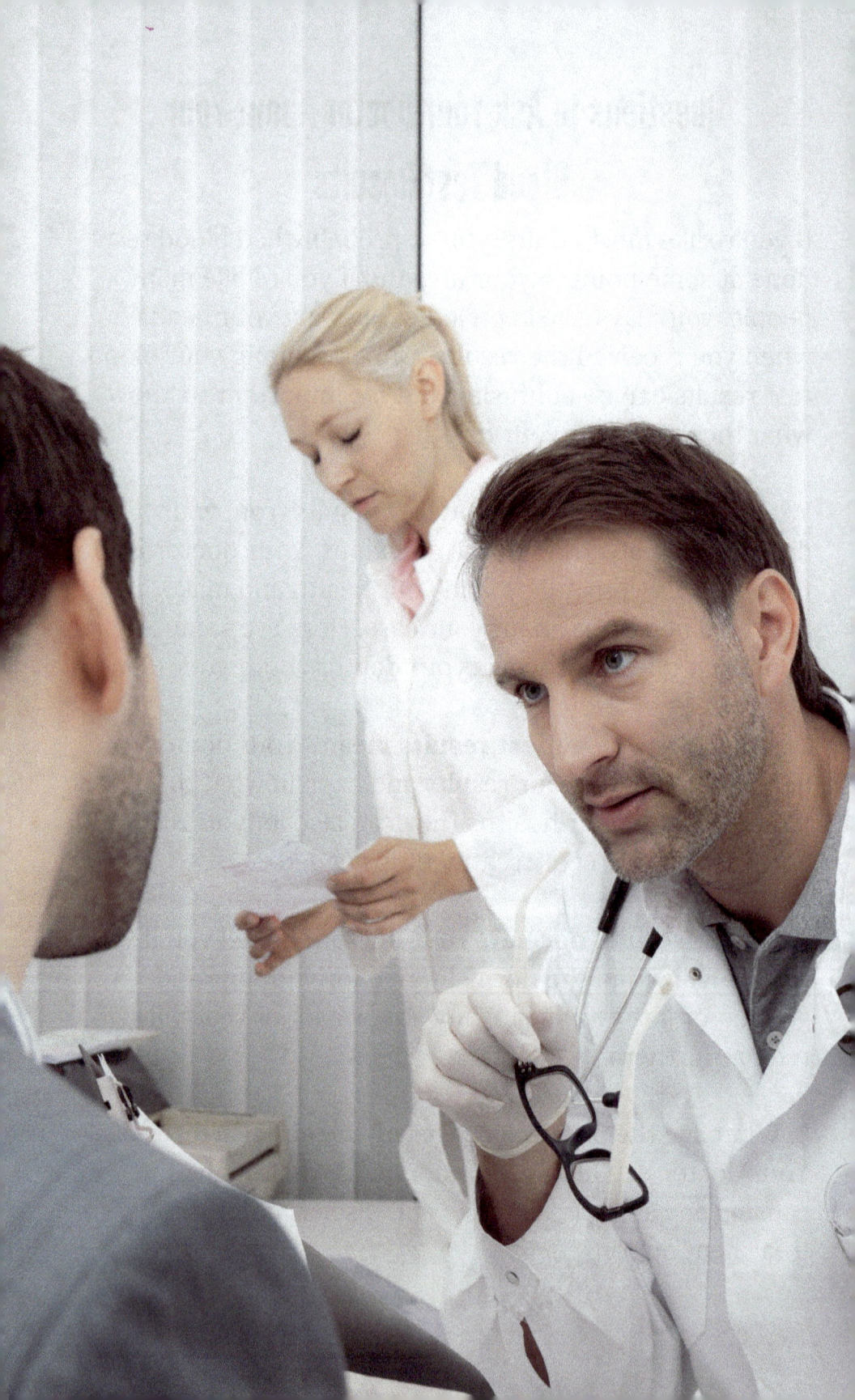

4. Are there any lifestyle changes I can make to improve my results? Your doctor can provide guidance on diet, exercise, and other lifestyle factors that may help improve your blood test results.

5. How often should I have blood tests done? Your doctor can recommend how often you should have blood tests done based on your age, medical history, and risk factors. Remember, it's important to advocate for your own health by asking questions and seeking clarification about your blood test results. By being proactive and informed, you can take control of your health and make the best decisions for your well-being.

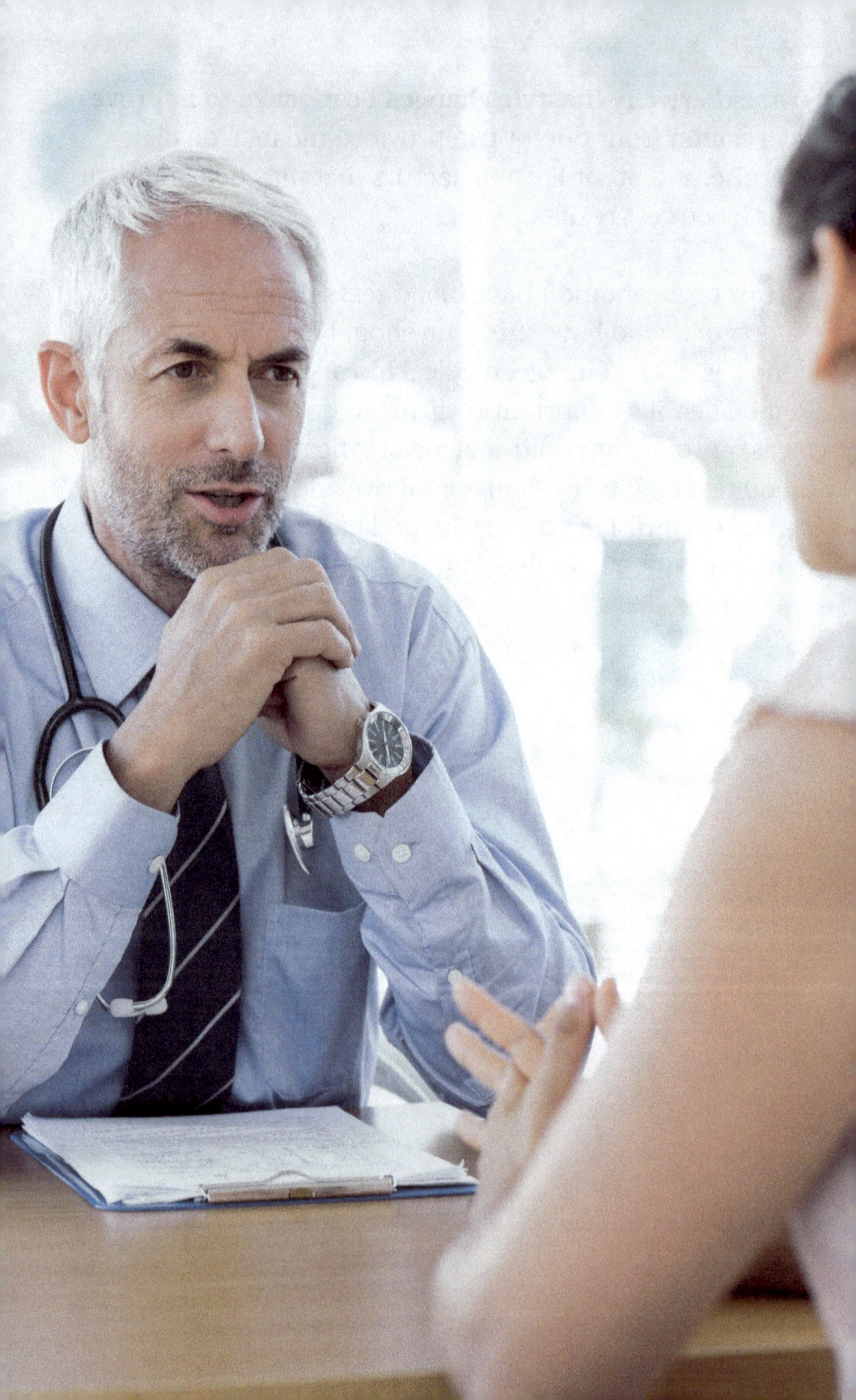

How to Advocate for Yourself in Healthcare Settings

Advocating for yourself in healthcare settings is crucial to ensuring you receive the best possible care and understanding of your medical results. This is especially important when it comes to interpreting your blood test results, as they can provide valuable insights into your overall health.

One of the first steps in advocating for yourself is to educate yourself about the different types of blood tests and what they measure. By understanding the purpose of each test, you can ask informed questions and have a better grasp of your results when they come back. When discussing your blood test results with your healthcare provider, don't be afraid to ask for clarification on anything you don't understand. It's important to advocate for yourself by making sure you have a clear understanding of what the results mean for your health and any potential next steps.

Additionally, if you have concerns about your blood test results or feel that something is not being addressed, don't hesitate to speak up. Your healthcare provider is there to help you, and it's important to advocate for yourself by expressing any concerns or questions you may have.

Another important aspect of advocating for yourself in healthcare settings is being proactive about your health. This includes following up on any recommended treatments or lifestyle changes based on your blood test

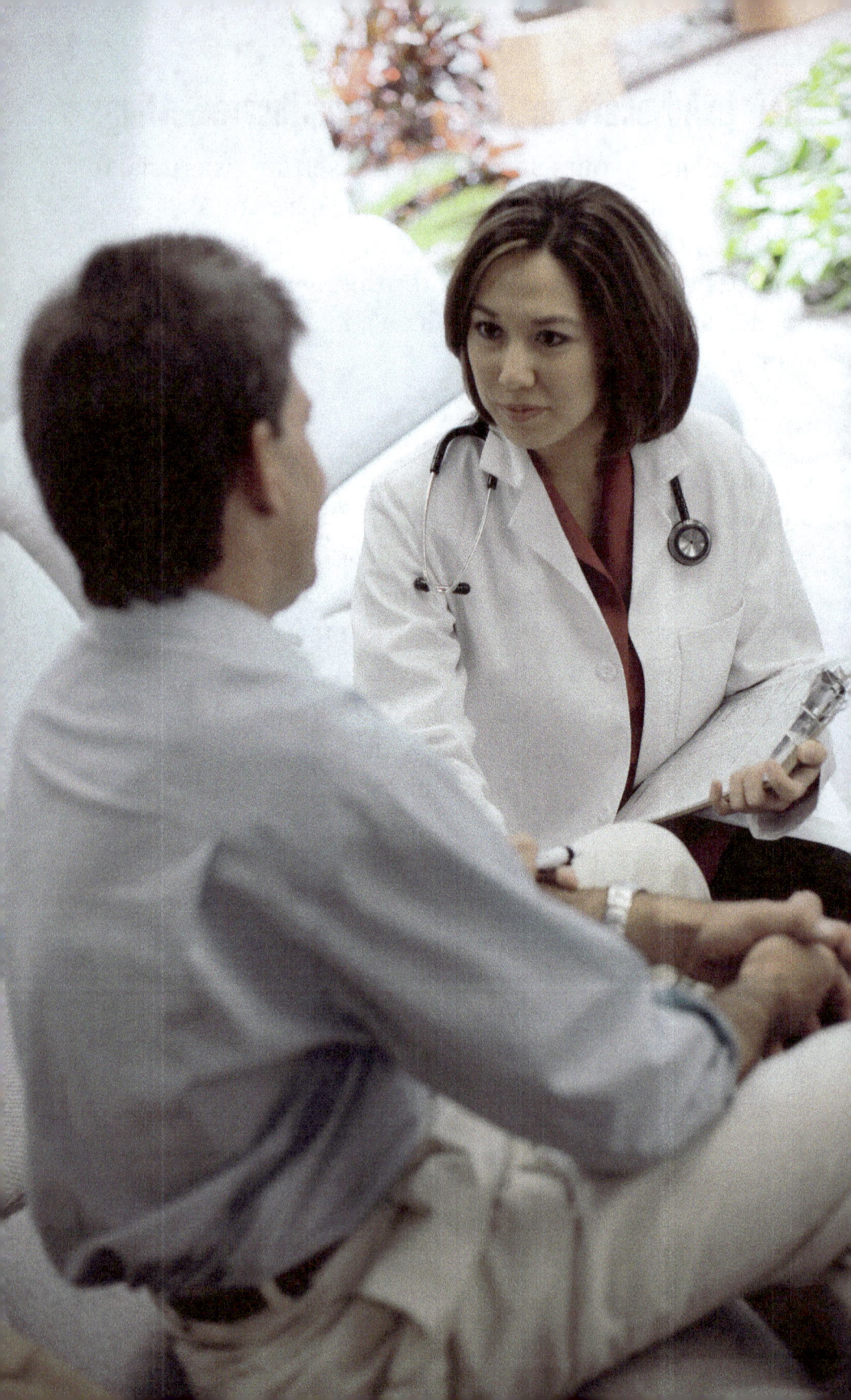

results, as well as scheduling regular check-ups to monitor your progress.

Overall, advocating for yourself in healthcare settings is essential for understanding your blood test results and ensuring you receive the best possible care. By educating yourself, asking questions, expressing concerns, and being proactive about your health, you can take control of your well-being and make informed decisions about your healthcare.

Seeking a Second Opinion

As adults, it is important to take charge of our health and be proactive in understanding our medical tests, especially when it comes to blood tests. One important aspect of advocating for your health is seeking a second opinion when necessary.

When you receive your blood test results, it is crucial to remember that they are not set in stone. Medical professionals are human and can make mistakes, and lab results can sometimes be misinterpreted. If you have any doubts or concerns about your results, don't be afraid to seek a second opinion.

There are several reasons why you might want to seek a second opinion on your blood test results. It could be that you don't understand the results or that they seem abnormal compared to your usual health status. In some cases, a second opinion can provide a fresh perspective and help you make more informed decisions about your health.

When seeking a second opinion, it is important to find a qualified and experienced healthcare professional who specializes in interpreting blood tests. This could be another doctor, a hematologist, or a specialist in the specific area of concern. Be sure to bring a copy of your original test results and any relevant medical history to your appointment.

Remember, your health is in your hands, and seeking a

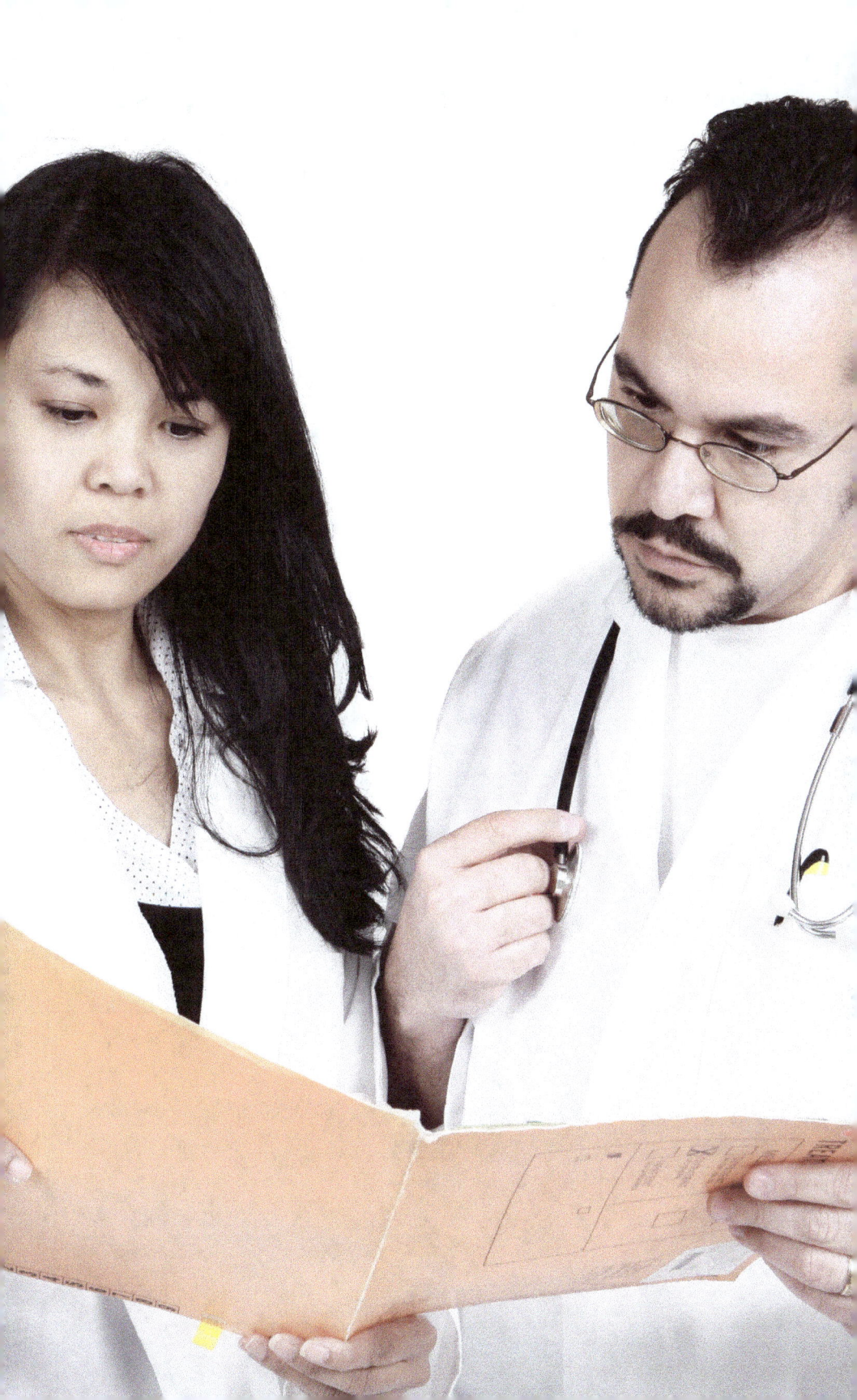

second opinion is your right as a patient. Don't hesitate to advocate for yourself and ensure that you fully understand your blood test results. By seeking a second opinion, you can gain peace of mind and make more informed decisions about your health.

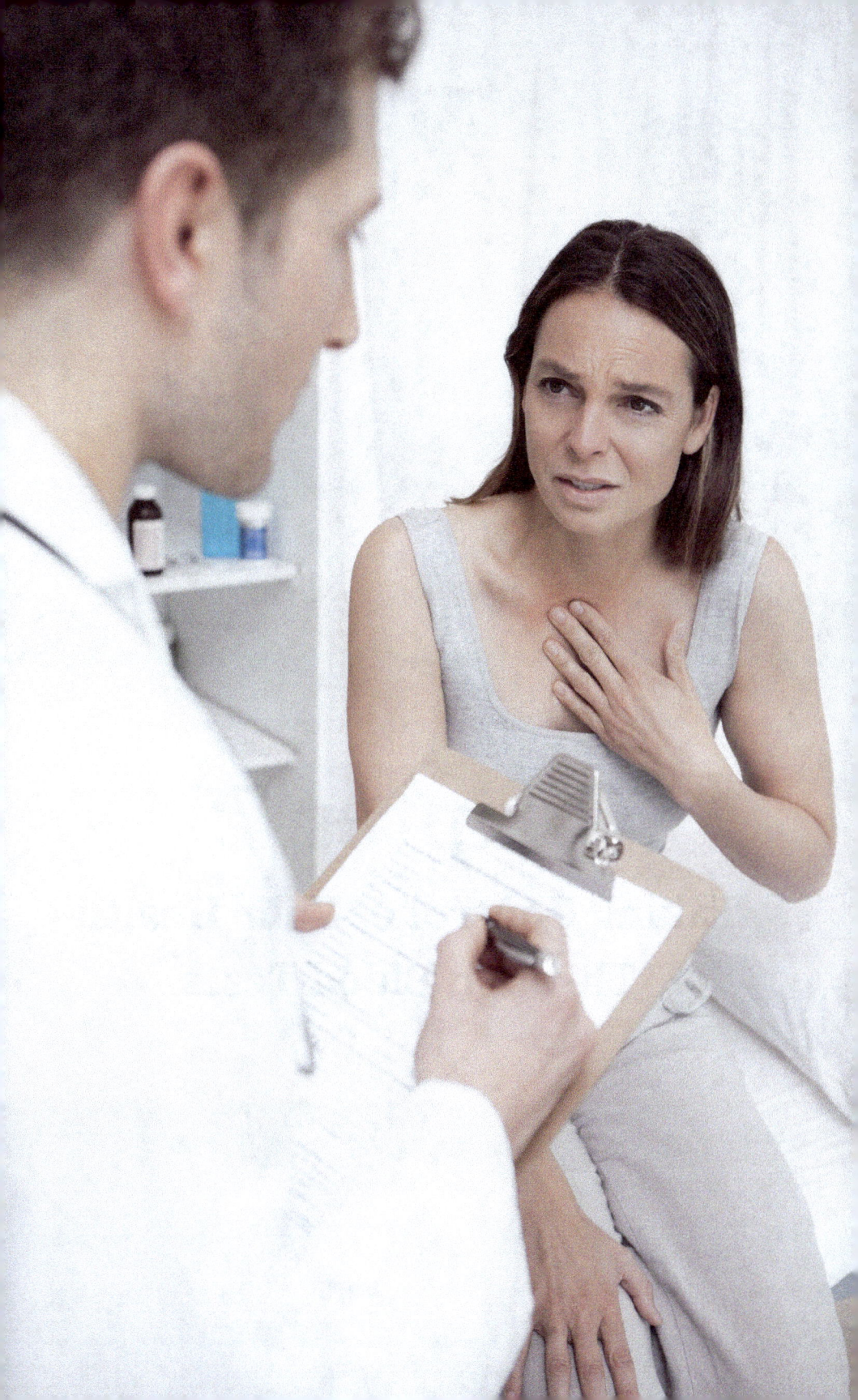

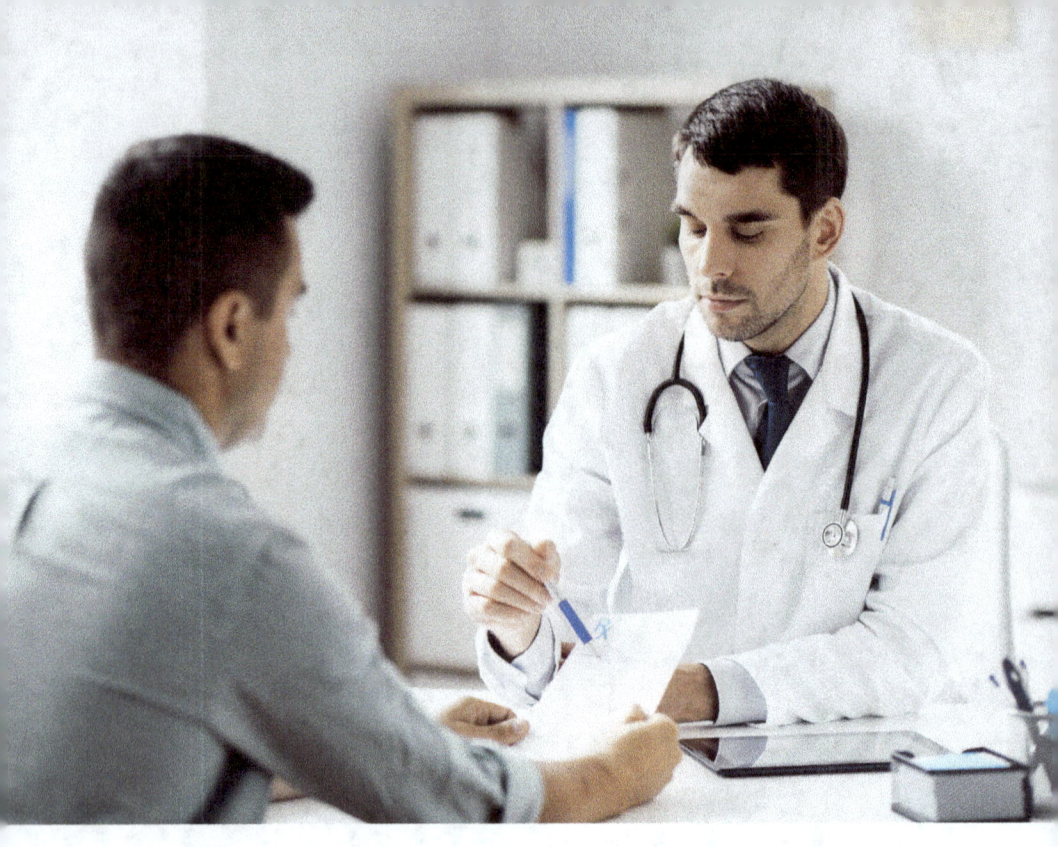

Chapter 7:

Taking Control of Your Health Through Blood Tests

Using Blood Tests to Monitor Chronic Conditions

Blood tests are an essential tool in monitoring chronic conditions such as diabetes, hypertension, and heart disease. These tests provide valuable information about your overall health and help your healthcare provider make informed decisions about your treatment plan.

One of the most common uses of blood tests in monitoring chronic conditions is to measure blood glucose levels in patients with diabetes. By regularly monitoring your blood sugar levels, you and your healthcare provider can work together to adjust your medication, diet, and lifestyle to keep your diabetes under control and prevent complications.

Blood tests can also help monitor conditions like hypertension by measuring levels of cholesterol, triglycerides, and other markers of heart health. By keeping track of these levels over time, you and your doctor can identify trends and make changes to your treatment plan as needed to reduce your risk of heart disease and stroke.

For individuals with chronic conditions such as autoimmune disorders or thyroid disease, blood tests can help monitor the progression of the disease and the effectiveness of treatment. By regularly checking levels of specific antibodies or hormones, your healthcare provider can make adjustments to your medication or recommend additional tests or treatments to manage your condition.

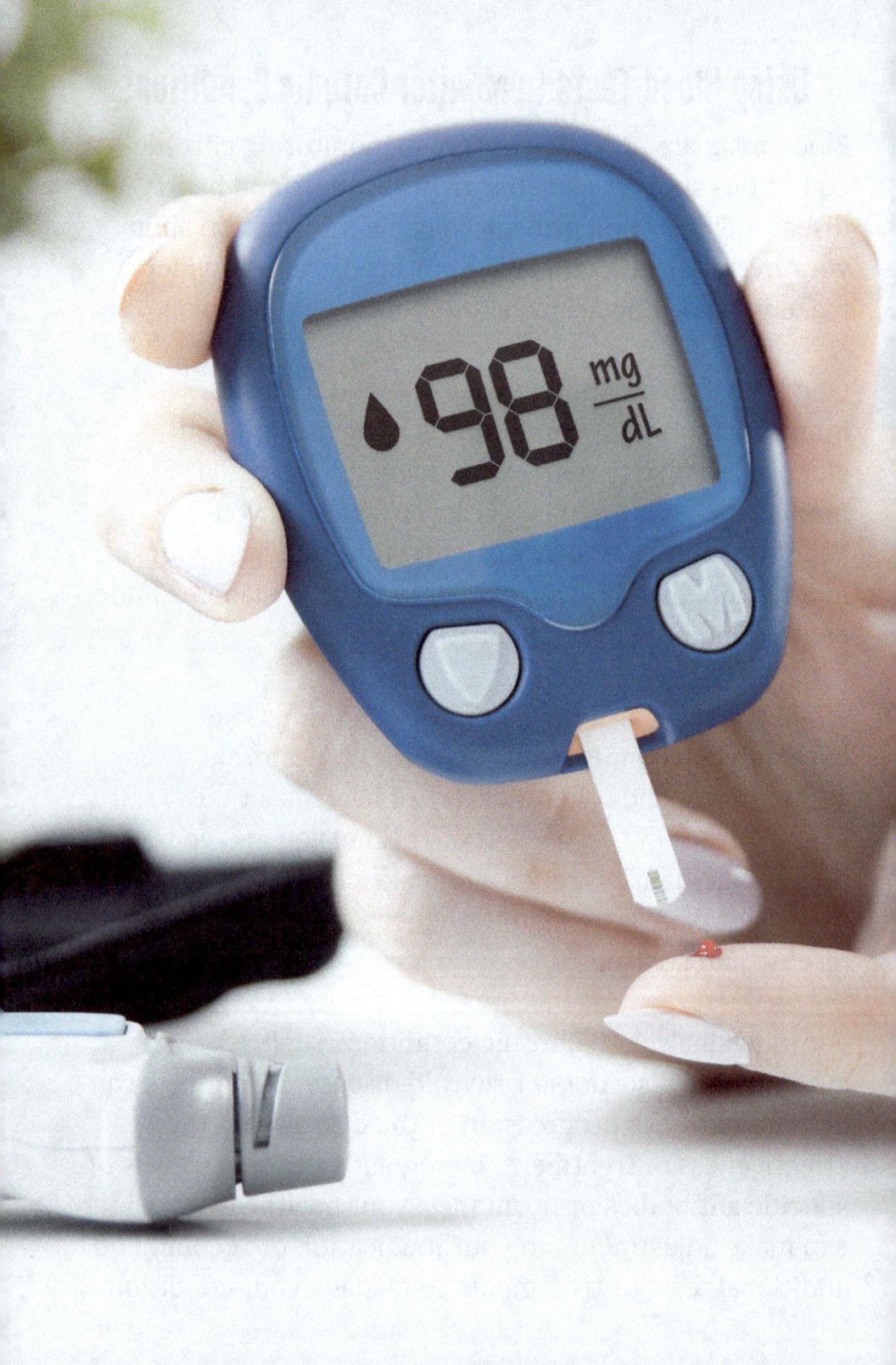

Overall, using blood tests to monitor chronic conditions is an important part of managing your health and preventing complications. By working closely with your healthcare provider and understanding the results of your blood tests, you can take an active role in managing your chronic condition and maintaining your overall well-being.

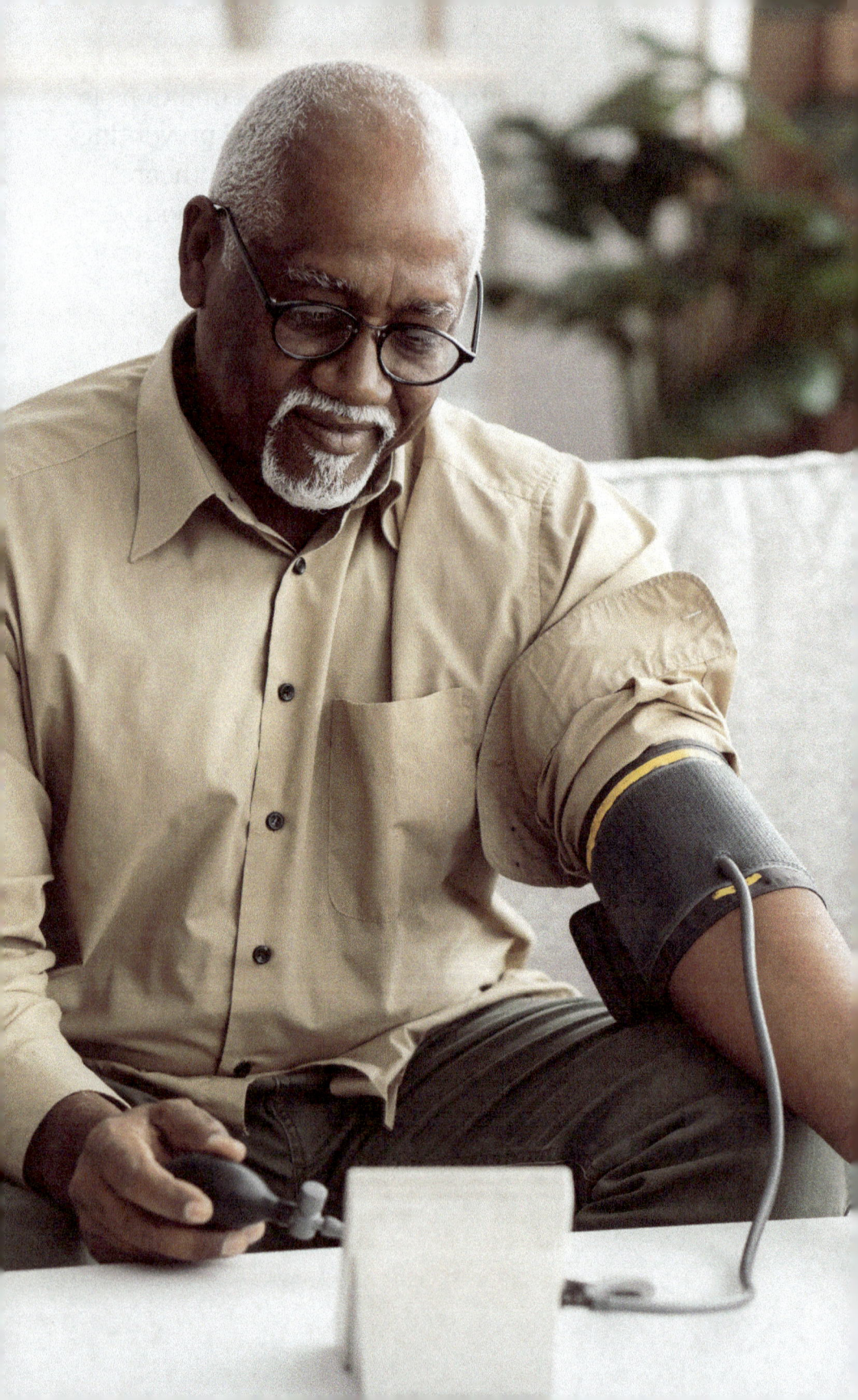

Preventative Health Screening with Blood Tests

Regular blood tests are a crucial component of preventative health screening, allowing healthcare providers to detect potential health issues before they escalate into more serious conditions. By understanding the results of these tests, adults can take proactive steps to maintain their well-being and make informed decisions about their health.

One common blood test used in preventative health screening is the complete blood count (CBC), which provides valuable information about red blood cells, white blood cells, and platelets. Abnormalities in these levels can indicate conditions such as anemia, infection, or blood disorders. By monitoring these levels through regular CBC tests, individuals can catch these issues early and work with their healthcare providers to address them.

Another important blood test for preventative health screening is the lipid panel, which measures cholesterol levels in the blood. High cholesterol levels can increase the risk of heart disease and stroke, making regular lipid panels essential for monitoring cardiovascular health. Understanding the results of a lipid panel can help individuals make dietary and lifestyle changes to improve their heart health.

Additionally, blood tests can screen for conditions such as diabetes, thyroid disorders, and liver function abnormalities. By staying up to date on these tests and

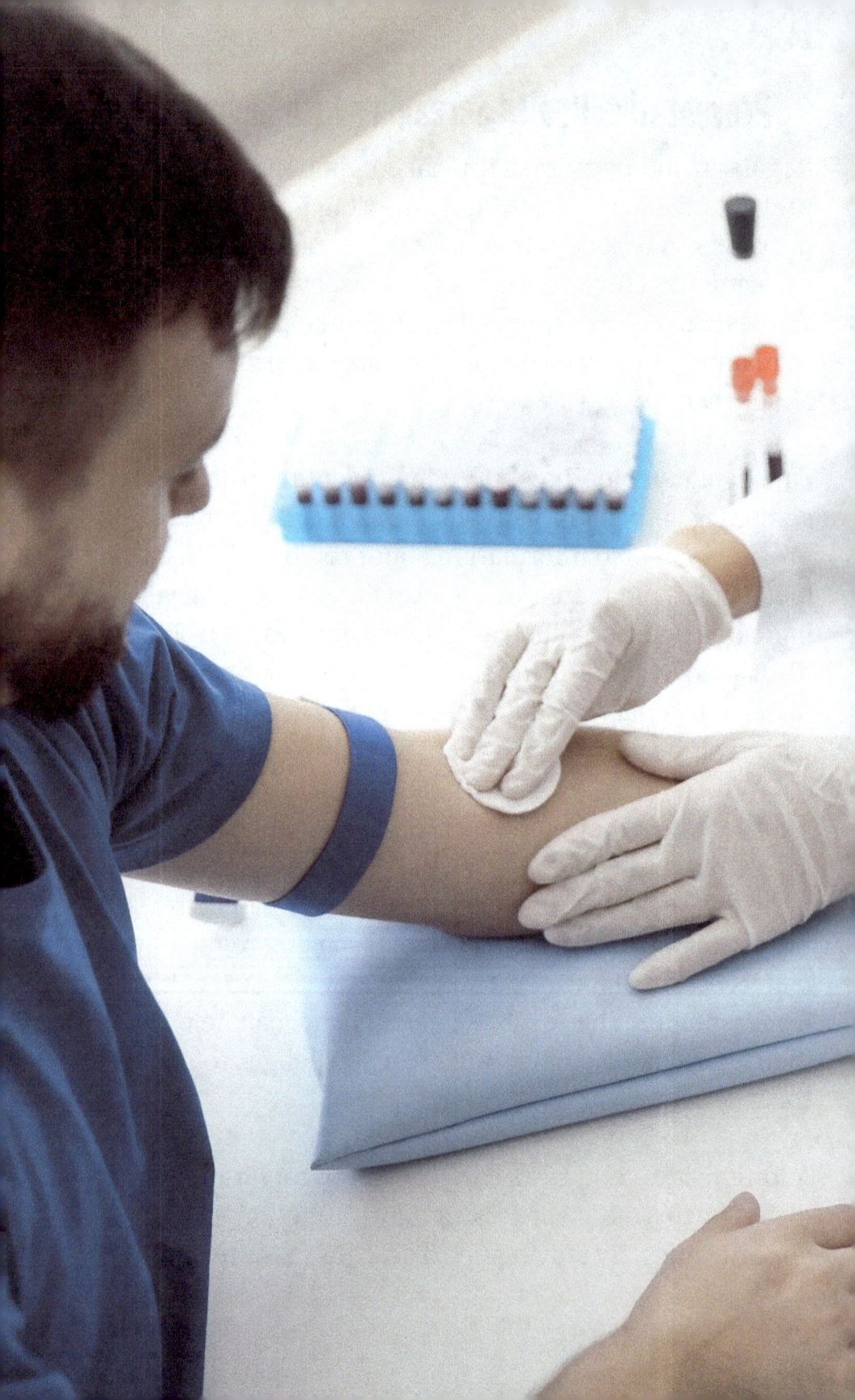

understanding their results, adults can take control of their health and work towards preventing serious health complications.

In conclusion, preventative health screening with blood tests is a powerful tool for maintaining overall well-being. By understanding the importance of these tests and the information they provide, adults can make informed decisions about their health and work towards a healthier future.

Lifestyle Changes Based on Blood Test Results

When it comes to understanding your blood test results, it's important to realize that they can provide valuable insights into your overall health and well-being. One of the key aspects of interpreting these results is understanding how they can inform lifestyle changes that may be necessary to improve your health.

Upon receiving your blood test results, it's essential to review them with your healthcare provider to gain a comprehensive understanding of what they mean for your health. Based on these results, your healthcare provider may recommend specific lifestyle changes that can help you achieve optimal health.

For example, if your blood test results show high levels of cholesterol, your healthcare provider may recommend dietary changes, such as reducing your intake of saturated fats and increasing your intake of fruits, vegetables, and whole grains. They may also suggest incorporating regular exercise into your routine to help lower cholesterol levels.

Similarly, if your blood test results indicate high blood sugar levels, your healthcare provider may recommend dietary changes, such as reducing your intake of sugary foods and beverages, and increasing your consumption of fiber-rich foods. Regular exercise and weight management may also be recommended to help stabilize blood sugar levels.

By understanding your blood test results and the lifestyle

Diet Plan

	Lunch	
		Dinner

changes that may be necessary based on these results, you can take proactive steps to improve your health and well-being. It's important to work closely with your healthcare provider to develop a personalized plan that addresses your specific needs and goals. Remember, small changes can lead to significant improvements in your overall health, so don't hesitate to take action based on your blood test results.

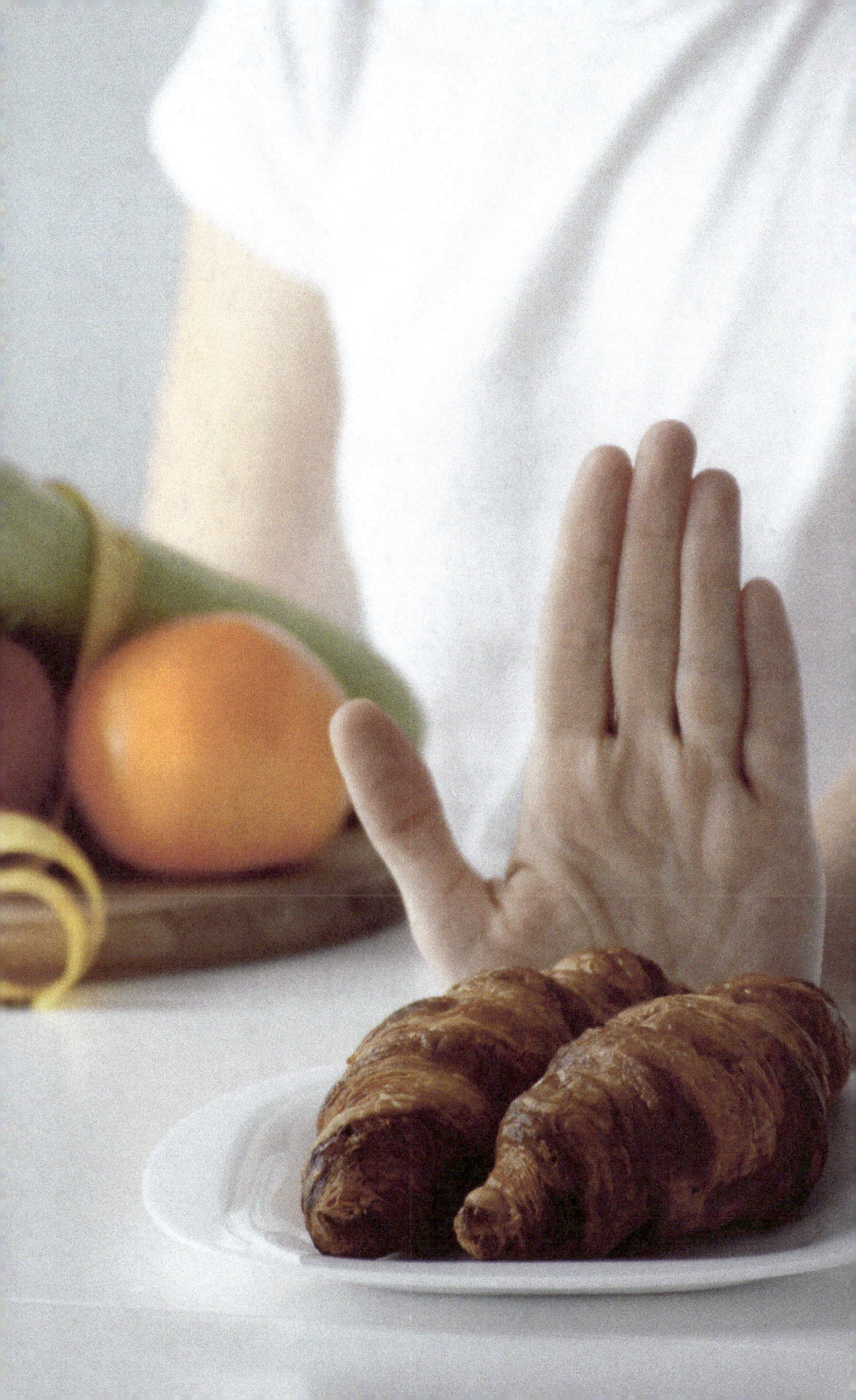

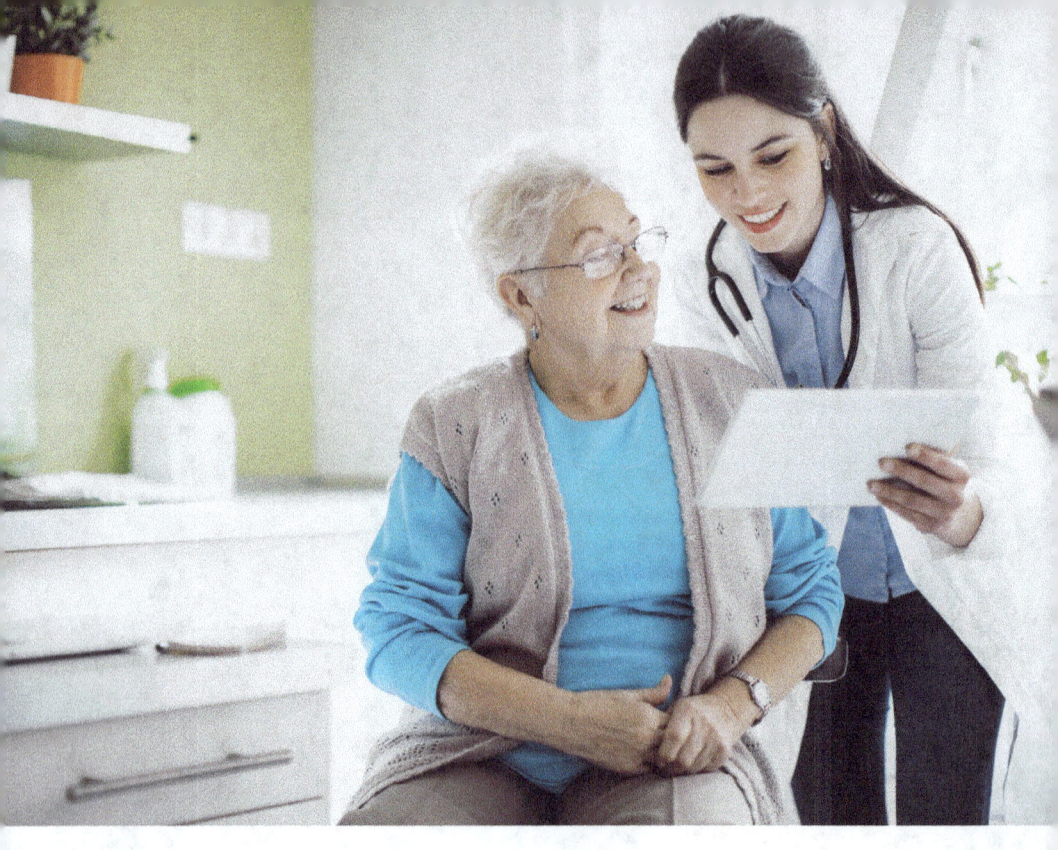

Chapter 8:

The Empowerment of Understanding

The Empowerment of Understanding Your Blood Test Results

Understanding your blood test results can be a powerful tool in taking control of your health and well-being. By gaining insight into what those numbers mean, you can make informed decisions about your lifestyle, diet, and medical treatment.

One of the first steps in interpreting your blood test results is understanding the basic components of a typical blood panel. This may include measurements of red blood cells, white blood cells, platelets, cholesterol levels, and various other markers that can provide valuable information about your overall health.

It's important to remember that blood test results are not just numbers on a page – they are a reflection of your body's internal workings. By understanding what each result means, you can detect potential health issues early on and take steps to address them before they become serious.

For example, elevated cholesterol levels may indicate a risk of heart disease, while low red blood cell counts could be a sign of anemia. By working with your healthcare provider to interpret these results, you can develop a plan to improve your health and prevent future complications. Empower yourself by asking questions and seeking clarification on any results that you don't understand. Your healthcare provider is there to help you make sense of your blood test results and provide guidance on how to improve your health outcomes. Ultimately, the empowerment that comes from understanding your blood test results can lead to better health outcomes and a higher quality of life. So take charge of your health today by diving into the world of blood test results and unlocking the potential for a healthier future.

Resources for Further Information on Blood Tests

For adults who want to delve deeper into understanding their blood tests, there are a plethora of resources available to help you navigate the complexities of medical results. Whether you are seeking information on specific tests, interpreting your results, or simply wanting to educate yourself further on the topic, the following resources can be invaluable in your journey to better understanding your health.

1. Websites: Websites such as Lab Tests Online (labtestsonline.org) provide detailed explanations of various blood tests, their purposes, and what the results may indicate. This user-friendly resource offers a wealth of information in an easy-to-understand format.

2. Books: There are several books available that delve into the world of blood tests and medical results. "The Patient's Guide to Medical Tests" by Joseph C. Segen and "Understanding Laboratory Tests: A Quick Reference" by Marjorie Schaub Di Lorenzo are highly recommended for those looking to expand their knowledge on the subject.

3. Healthcare Providers: Your healthcare provider is an invaluable resource when it comes to understanding your blood tests. Don't hesitate to ask questions and seek clarification on any aspect of your results that you may not fully grasp.

4. Support Groups: Joining a support group or online forum for individuals who are also navigating the world of

blood tests can provide a sense of community and the opportunity to learn from others' experiences.

5. Online Courses: Platforms such as Coursera and Khan Academy offer free online courses on topics related to medical tests and laboratory results. These courses can provide a more in-depth understanding of the subject matter.

By utilizing these resources, you can empower yourself to take control of your health and make informed decisions based on your blood test results. Remember, knowledge is power, and the more you understand about your medical tests, the better equipped you will be to advocate for your own health and well-being.

Taking Charge of Your Health Through Knowledge

In order to truly take charge of your health, it is essential to have a solid understanding of your blood test results. Many adults receive their blood test results from their doctor without fully comprehending what the numbers and values actually mean. By educating yourself on how to interpret these results, you can gain valuable insight into your overall health and make informed decisions about your well-being.

One of the first steps in understanding your blood test results is to familiarize yourself with the common metrics that are measured in a standard blood test. These may include levels of white blood cells, red blood cells, platelets, cholesterol, glucose, and various other markers that can provide important information about your health. By learning about the normal ranges for these metrics, you can better understand whether your results fall within a healthy range or if there are any potential concerns that need to be addressed.

Additionally, it is important to understand the significance of trends in your blood test results over time. By tracking changes in your levels of various markers, you can identify patterns that may indicate the presence of an underlying health condition or the effectiveness of a particular treatment plan. This knowledge can empower you to work proactively with your healthcare provider to address any issues that may arise.

By taking charge of your health through knowledge, you

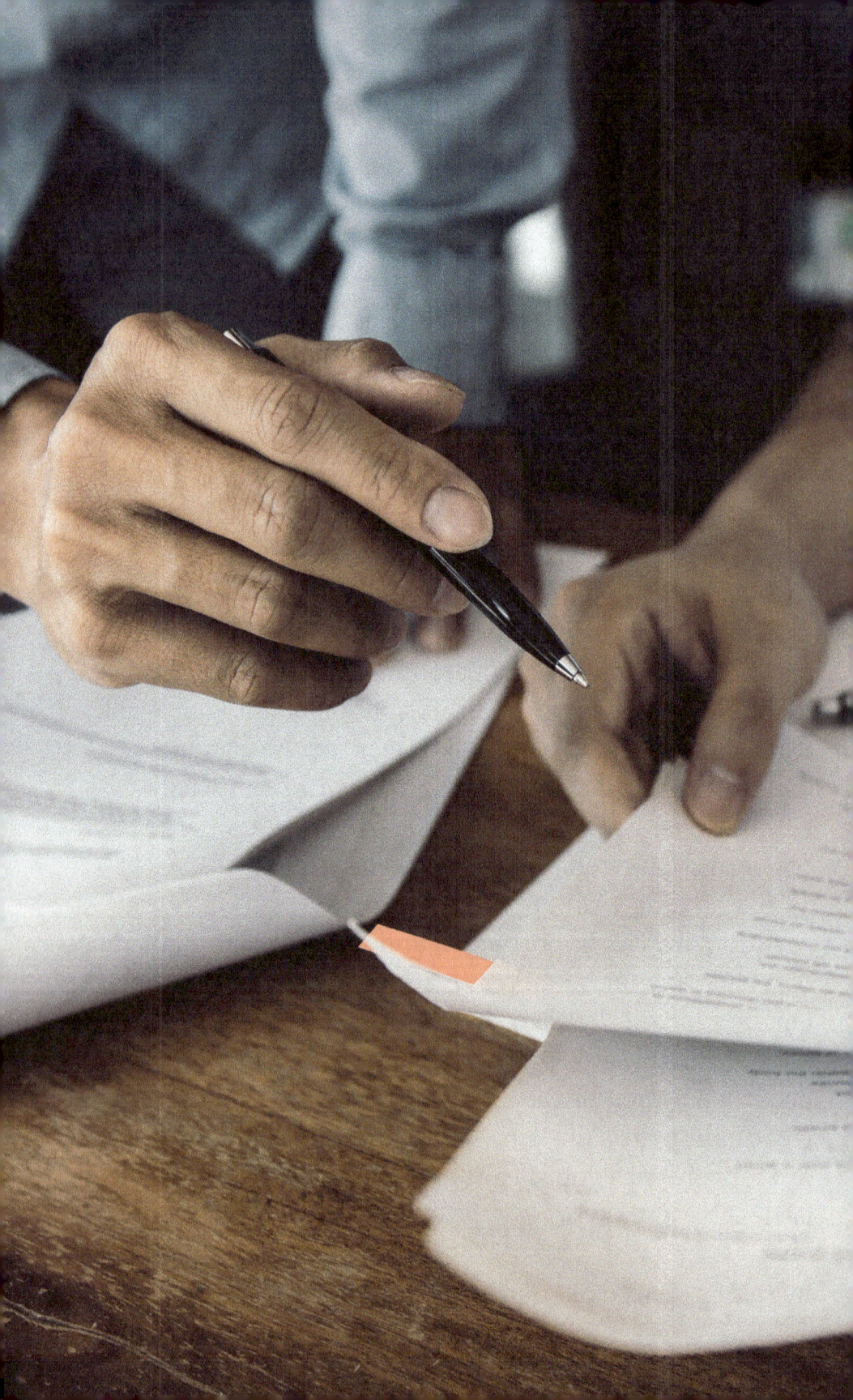

can become an active participant in your own healthcare journey. Armed with a better understanding of your blood test results, you can make informed decisions about your lifestyle, diet, and medical treatment options. Ultimately, being proactive and informed about your health can lead to better outcomes and a higher quality of life.

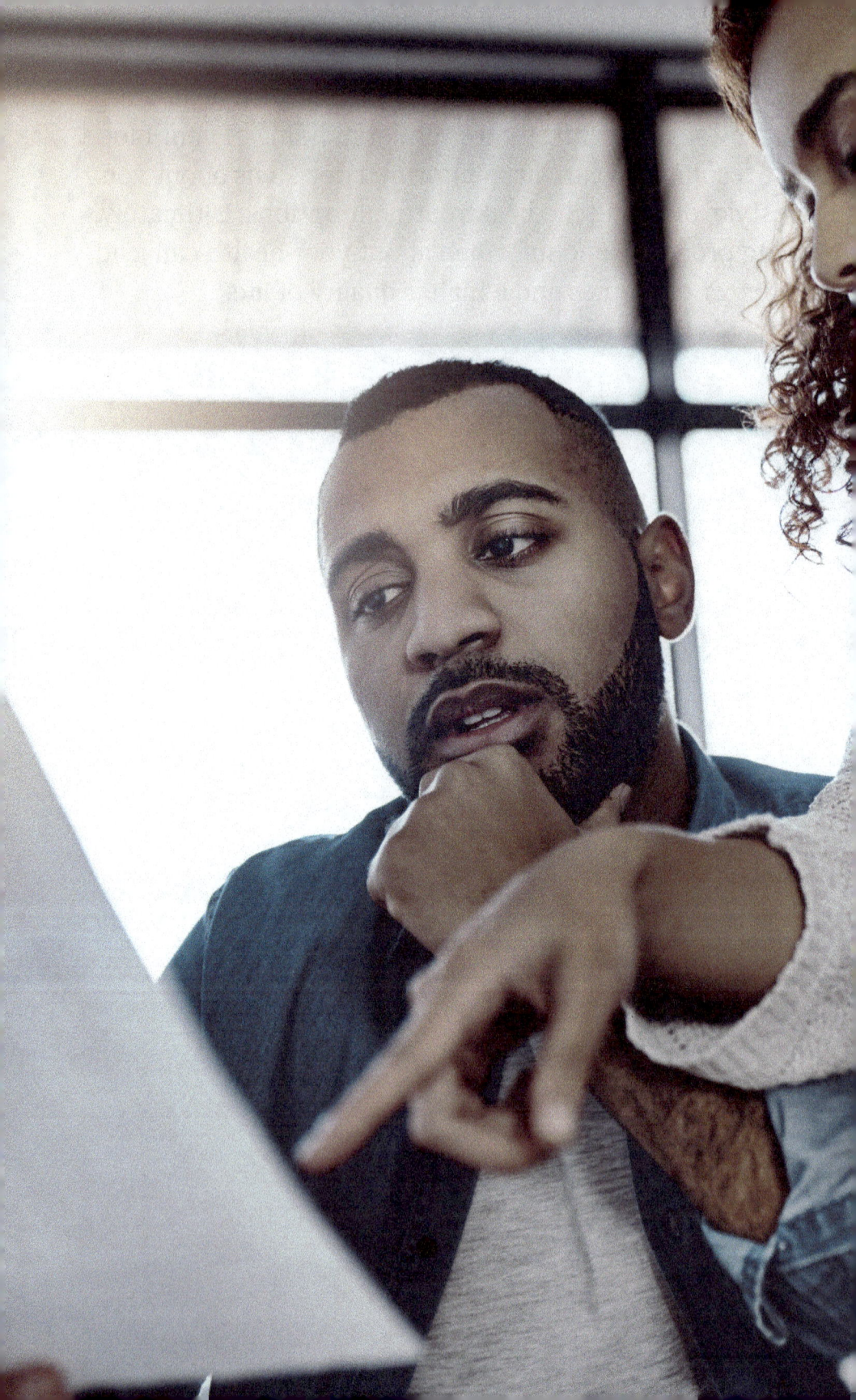